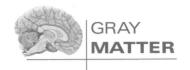
GRAY
MATTER

Pain

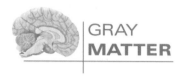

GRAY
MATTER

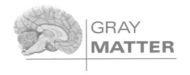
GRAY
MATTER

Pain

Bryan C. Hains, Ph.D.

Series Editor
Eric H. Chudler, Ph.D.

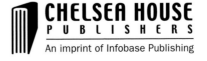

CHELSEA HOUSE
PUBLISHERS
An imprint of Infobase Publishing

Pain

Chelsea House
An imprint of Infobase Publishing
132 West 31st Street
New York, NY 10001

978-0-7910-8951-4

Library of Congress Cataloging-in-Publication Data

Hains, Bryan C.
  Pain / Bryan C. Hains.
    p. cm. —(Gray matter)
  Includes bibliographical references and index.
  ISBN 0-7910-8951-7 (hardcover)
  1. Pain—Juvenile literature. I. Title. II. Series.
  RB127.H324 2006
  616'.0472—dc22   2006015133

Chelsea House books are available at special discounts when purchased in bulk quantities for businesses, associations, institutions, or sales promotions. Please call our Special Sales Department in New York at (212) 967-8800 or (800) 322-8755.

You can find Chelsea House on the World Wide Web at http://www.chelseahouse.com

Series and cover design by Terry Mallon

Printed in the United States of America

Bang EJB 10 9 8 7 6 5 4 3 2 1

This book is printed on acid-free paper.

All links and Web addresses were checked and verified to be correct at the time of publication. Because of the dynamic nature of the Web, some addresses and links may have changed since publication and may no longer be valid.

Contents

1 | History of Sensation and Pain

Sensation is the way that the body receives information from its internal and external environments. The concept of such an interaction, and how it is produced, has evolved throughout recorded history. The ancient Greeks and Romans were the first to develop a theory of how the body sensed the world. They originated the idea that the central nervous system plays a role in producing perception, although the concept of the nervous system and its capabilities as we now think of it was not much developed at the time. Support for these early theories began to accumulate during the Renaissance with the discoveries of Leonardo da Vinci and others. These thinkers more precisely defined the role of the nervous system, including the **peripheral nerves**, **spinal cord**, and **brain**, as the key components of the nervous system responsible for sensation. A few hundred years later, in the seventeenth and eighteenth centuries, the study of how the body and senses relate to each other became a major topic of study among the world's most important philosopher-scientists.

In his book titled *Discourse on Method*, the French philosopher René Descartes hypothesized that the actions of animals could be explained entirely in terms of mechanical principles. To understand these principles, Descartes advocated the use of physiological research to uncover the mechanisms of sensation and pain. Through these methods, in his essay

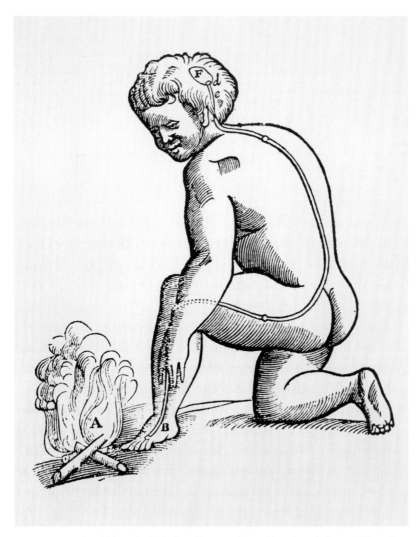

Figure 1.1 In this sketch by Descartes, the heat from the fire (*A*), starts a chain of processes that begins at the affected spot of the skin, (*B*), and continues up the nerve tube until a pore of a cavity, (*F*), is opened. Descartes believed that this opening allowed the animal spirits in the cavity to enter the nerve tube and eventually travel to the muscles that pull the foot from the fire. While the figure shows that Descartes anticipated the basic idea of reflex action, it also indicates that he did not realize the anatomical distinction between sensory and motor nerves.

"L'homme," he put forth the idea that "animal spirits" flowing through the nerves of animals functioned to produce reflex behaviors to painful stimuli (Figure 1.1). His theories of the reflex and of the ability to explain behavior mechanistically gave direction to future research.

As Descartes predicted, sensory systems receive information from the environment through specialized receptors and transmit this information to the central nervous system. In addition to receiving sensation from the outside world, we also receive information from within the body through receptors in **viscera**, muscles, joints, and blood vessels.

In the late 1800s, a physician and experimental psychologist named Hermann von Helmholtz advanced the idea that the skin's senses could be divided into several **modalities**. Helmholtz proposed that each stimulus was encoded by the peripheral nervous system, then decoded by the central nervous system to produce an experience. The central nervous system is the part of the nervous system that is made up of the brain and spinal cord, whereas the peripheral nervous system is made up of nerves and receptors in the body and extremities. We now know that all sensory pathways begin with a stimulus that acts on specialized sensory receptors that convert the stimulus into neural signals (a process called transduction) and transmit the signals via a sensory neuron to the brain, where they are interpreted. In perceiving a sensation, we transform it from a simple electrical impulse into the complex mental-emotional phenomenon called perception.

To create an accurate neural representation of sensory stimuli, the brain must distinguish four properties about a stimulus: its modality, intensity, duration, and location. The combination of these attributes gives rise to a sensation. Different forms of energy are transformed by receptors in the nervous system into readable signals. Each receptor type is activated by a particular type of stimulus. The brain then associates a signal coming in from a specific group of receptors with a specific modality. The sensory system is made up of a number of receptor types, each detecting a simple modality such as light, touch, heat, cold, or pain. This direct association between a receptor and its representation in the brain is called **labeled line** coding. In this way there is a direct connection between the stimulus and the corresponding part of the brain that interprets it.

The amount of a sensation experienced depends on the strength of the stimulus. The number of receptors activated, as well as the frequency of nerve firing in response to stimulation, define stimulus **intensity**. A certain stimulation intensity, or sensory threshold, is required for the active perception of a stimulus. The duration of a sensation is defined by the relationship between the stimulus intensity and the time in which it is perceived. The firing period of the **action potentials** conveys to the nervous system the duration of the stimulation. Finally, each sensory receptor is most sensitive to the stimulation of a specific area on the skin or in its end territory called a **receptive field**. When action potentials are generated in a sensory neuron, the neuron's receptive field codes the stimulus location. The receptive fields are organized in an orderly fashion into sensory areas within the brain to form sensory maps of the body.

WHAT IS PAIN?

According to the philosopher Aristotle, sight, sound, touch, smell, and taste are the primary ways in which the nervous system receives information about the environment. This classification schema is still used today. Aristotle, like many others, grouped together many submodalities of touch into one category. Scientists now consider the sensations of touch-pressure, flutter-vibration, tickle, warmth, cold, pain, itch, position sense, and sense of movement to be separate modalities that do not exclusively belong to touch. Warmth and cold, for example, do not require skin contact like touch. Some of these sensations can be even further divided, especially those related to pain sensation. For example, pain can include stabbing pain, cramping pain, and/or burning pain.

The International Association for the Study of Pain defines pain as an unpleasant sensory and emotional experience associated with actual or potential tissue damage, or described in terms of such damage. The function of pain is thought to be threefold: First, in the short term, pain causes us to withdraw from some source that is causing the pain, preventing damage to the body. Second, long-term pain promotes behaviors that promote recovery from injury, such as inactivity, grooming, and eating and drinking. Third, the vocal expression of pain serves as a social signal to other animals. Producing a scream or yelp after experiencing a painful stimulus may have an adaptive value by communicating the potential harm to others that are nearby, or eliciting caregiving behavior from others after injury.

Pain is so common that we easily forget its purpose: The experience of pain leads to behaviors that remove the body from a source of harm. This is proven by the fact that a rare genetic insensitivity to pain can result in bodily damage that can lead to death. Case histories reveal that the bodies of people who cannot feel pain show extensive damage and scarring from injuries to fingers, hands, and legs. The first reported person with **congenital insensitivity to pain** worked as a "human pincushion" in a carnival. Congenital insensitivity to pain is a rare inherited disorder usually manifested in childhood by a history of unexplained injury, indifference to pain stimuli, or self-mutilation. This disorder results in the absence of normal responses to sensations of pain, heat, and cold, and is caused by a genetic mutation that prevents the formation of nerve cells that are responsible for transmitting pain signals to the brain.

One boy with pain insensitivity who worked on a sugar cane plantation would accidentally cut the front of his shins with his machete while chopping sugar cane. Repeated injuries caused severe infection of his legs that resulted in a systemic blood infection and death. If he had been aware of his injuries and infection through the sensation of pain, treatment might have saved his life.

Many people with this disorder die young, frequently from trauma to the body. These cases suggest that pain guides adaptive behavior by indicating potential and ongoing harm to the body.

THE EXPERIENCE OF PAIN

Pain is always subjective, and for this reason it is difficult to define precisely (Figure 1.2). Each individual learns the meaning of pain through experiences related to injury in early life. It is unquestionably a sensation of the body, but it is also always unpleasant and therefore also an emotional experience. Learning, experience, emotion, gender, age, and culture all shape the experience of pain. In other words, we experience pain as we interpret it. In 1937, the surgeon René Leriche aptly noted that pain always contains at its heart the human encounter with meaning. Our brains perceive pain, and our intellect and emotions register its depth, source, and implications. People can also report pain in the absence of tissue damage or disease; this usually happens for psychological reasons. There is no way to distinguish this experience of pain from that associated with real damage, and all pain must be treated as real.

The intensity of a given stimulus that produces pain is variable from person to person, and a distinction must be made between an individual's **pain threshold** and **pain tolerance**. The pain threshold, like other sensory thresholds, is a hard-wired feature of the nervous system. It is a measure of the least

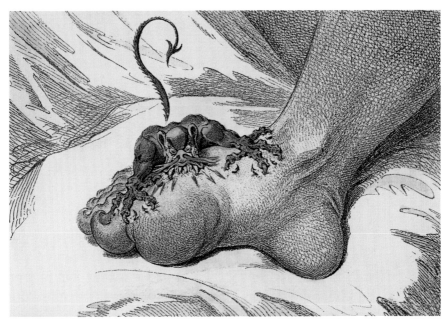

Figure 1.2 Gout is a recurrent disease characterized by painful inflammation of the joints. In his painting "The Gout" (1799), James Gillray illustrates the painfully affected joint of the big toe as a demon with a pointed tail attacking its victim with sharp fangs and claws.

amount of stimulation that elicits the sensation of pain. For mechanical stimuli, the difference between a low-intensity press and higher-intensity pinching of the skin can cause pain. With thermal stimulation, the skin temperature threshold that must be met to elicit the sensation of burning is 45°C (113°F). Pain tolerance is defined as the amount of pain a subject can withstand, and it varies enormously. This is difficult to test or define, and makes comparison of pain tolerance between individuals complicated.

■ Learn more about the contents of this chapter   Search the Internet for *International Association for the Study of Pain*, *history of pain*, and *congenital insensitivity to pain*.

2 | Skin and the Periphery

We receive information about our surroundings through highly specialized sensory structures in our skin and peripheral tissues. Our biological sensors can detect and interpret exquisite differences in touch, temperature, vibration, pressure, stretch, sound, light, odor, taste, and other forms of information. Signals from these receptors are converted to electrical impulses and communicated through peripheral nerves to the spinal cord, where they undergo further processing before being relayed to the brain.

SKIN AND RECEPTORS

The body has four different types of skin, each of which serves a different biological function. Mucous membrane is a layer of skin that surrounds the inner lining of the mouth, nose, and bodily orifices. Mucocutaneous skin forms the boundary skin between the mucous membrane and hairy skin, lips, and tongue. The skin types most commonly thought of are glabrous and hairy skin. **Glabrous** skin has no hair, such as that on the soles of the hands and feet. Hairy skin has hair follicles and is covered with hair. The skin is one of a number of complex multicellular structures specialized to detect one particular class of stimuli, as well as to protect the body from infection, among other functions.

Embedded within the skin are specialized sensory receptors that respond to particular types of stimuli from the external world and convert this information into electrical signals that the nervous system uses to relay messages, called action potentials. The transformation of one energy source, such as light or touch, to another, such as an action potential, is called **sensory transduction**. Signal transduction is performed by the endings of nerve fibers called **sensory receptors**, specialized detectors for a particular type of stimulus.

Sensory receptors convert external stimuli into action potentials much like a microphone picks up sound waves and converts them into electrical signals that are received and amplified by a loudspeaker. Similar to a microphone that is specialized in regard to the type of signal it can detect, convert, and relay, sensory receptors are tuned to respond to precise types of stimuli.

Receptive fields are territories of the skin where individual sensory neurons are responsive to stimuli. A neuron's receptive field can vary in size depending on how sensitive the neuron needs to be in detecting a stimulus. Receptive fields located on highly sensitive areas of the body such as the fingers and lips are very small, whereas receptive fields of neurons that **innervate** the palm or forehead are larger. The largest receptive fields are found on the back of the body. As a general rule, more precise sensation requires smaller receptive fields on individual receptors, as well as a higher density of receptors.

The receptive field determines spatial resolution, i.e., the number of points that can be detected in a given area of skin. This translates into how finely responsive the receptor is, and limits the resolution of the neuron, which is known as **tactile resolution**. For example, the palm might not be able to distinguish between the width of a pencil and a piece of chalk because receptive fields of individual receptors are larger, and the density of receptive fields is lower, than in the fingertips. The fine

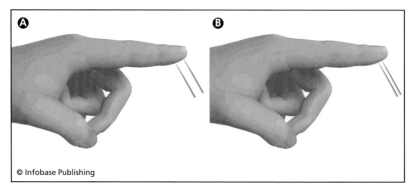

© Infobase Publishing

Figure 2.1 In figure A, the patient can sense the pressure of two distinct wooden sticks. When the sticks are brought closer together, as in figure B, the patient feels as though only one stick is being pressed against the skin.

touch system permits the discrimination between two points on the skin that are very close together, and thus, between small objects or subtle differences in the texture of an object. Tactile resolution can vary by 20-fold from the back of the body to the fingertip (Figure 2.1).

Skin receptors are divided into classes based on their functions: (1) mechanoreceptors, which respond to touch and pressure; (2) nociceptors, which respond to painful stimuli; (3) thermoreceptors; which respond to hot and cold stimuli; and (4) chemoreceptors, which respond to certain chemicals.

MECHANORECEPTORS

Mechanoreceptors of glabrous and hairy skin receive and transmit information to the central nervous system regarding light touch and pressure. They are specialized receptors at the ending of nerve fibers that contain mechanosensitive ion channels, whose activation can be altered by mechanical force. Ion channels are holes in cell membranes that regulate the flow of Na, K, Cl, and Ca into the cell which cause changes in membrane potential and depolarization. Mechanical stress is subsequently transformed into an electrical response as the ion channel opens its pore and the receptor depolarizes, or fires. Features of mechanoreceptors, such as the size of the receptive field and the temporal response (how rapidly or slowly it adapts to an ongoing stimulus) are dependent on how the nerve ending is wired into its surrounding end capsule. Distinctly different types of mechanoreceptors exist based on the nature of the stimulus that they respond to.

Pacinian corpuscles respond to touch, pressure, vibration, or any other kind of mechanical stimulus that causes a deformation of the shape of the corpuscle. They are located in the deeper layer of the skin called the dermis, and have the appearance of an onion. Pacinian corpuscles are made up of 20–70 concentric fluid-separated wrappings of connective tissue. Each Pacinian corpuscle is attached to a single nerve fiber that is covered by a sensitive membrane covered in sodium ion channels. In its resting state, the corpuscle is not compressed, and thus there is no deformation of the nerve ending or action potential. When the membrane is compressed, the nerve ending deforms and sodium channels are stretched open, causing the receptor to fire. Because there is some space between each corpuscle, after compression it moves slightly and resumes its normal shape. Pacinian corpuscles have receptive fields with a cross section that is one inch in diameter.

The Pacinian corpuscle is said to be rapidly adapting, meaning that at the onset of a stimulus the receptor undergoes a high rate of firing that ends quickly. When the corpuscle is initially stimulated it fires rapidly, but with continuous pressure, the corpuscle decreases the frequency of action potential generation. This process occurs in many sensory receptors and is called adaptation. It serves to reduce the amount of information being continuously sent to the brain. An example of adaptation occurs when we wear a wristwatch—initially we notice the watch and feel it on our wrists after putting it on, but over time we do not feel it there anymore and ignore it. The speed of adaptation is different among different types of receptors depending on their biological function.

In this regard, mechanoreceptors encode change in the environment. If there is no change in the intensity or nature of the stimulus, the receptor undergoes adaptation. But if the stimulus changes (such as when the watch is moved around on the wrist), a new train of action potentials will be produced. Adaptation serves to provide only key information to the brain, and to prevent bombardment with excess information.

Meissner's corpuscles are embedded within epidermal ridges, have very small receptive fields, and are rapidly adapting. Only one-tenth the size of Pacinian corpuscles, they are located in high density in locations of the greatest sensitivity (such as the fingertips) and are thus fine touch and vibration receptors. Meissner's corpuscles are encapsulated receptors, surrounded by concentric layers of connective tissue.

Pacinian and Meissner's corpuscles are similar in function, but relay different types of information to the brain. For example, if an unknown object is placed in the hand, Pacinian corpuscles will transmit information regarding its weight, overall shape, and size, while Meissner's corpuscles will transmit information regarding its fine features such as edges, texture, and detail. The combination of these two unique streams of information allows the brain to identify the object.

Ruffini endings respond to stretching of the skin. They are found in the deeper dermal skin layer, primarily of the palms of the hands and the soles of the feet. Their structure resembles a spindle that forms a thin fluid-filled capsule that is oriented parallel to the surface of the skin. Capsules of Ruffini endings have bundles of a connective tissue meshwork that anchor the capsule to the surrounding tissue and contain nerve fibers of the **afferent** (incoming) nerve. They respond to tension in the surrounding collagen fibers. Ruffini endings have large receptive fields, and are slowly adapting.

Merkel's disks are touch receptors that primarily help to distinguish the shapes of objects, edges, and rough texture. They are located in the topmost layer of skin called the epidermis, particularly in the thick skin of the palms and soles. They are found in high density within the fingertips and lips, and make up about 25 percent of all mechanoreceptors. Merkel's disks are each associated with individual nerve fibers that enlarge into a disk-shaped nerve ending that resides in close proximity to another specialized cell. At this synapse-like junction, neurotransmitter molecules that signal between receptors and neurons are released onto the Merkel's disk when stimulated. Merkel's disks have small receptive fields and are slowly adapting.

NOCICEPTORS AND THERMORECEPTORS

Nociceptors are relatively less specialized nerve endings that transmit information about stimuli that threaten or damage the body (Figure 2.2). They are also active when damage is underway, but their function is preventative in that they are designed to protect the body from damage. In this regard, pain signals produced by nociceptors are a good thing when experienced in their proper context. The word nociception is derived from the Latin root *noci*, meaning "to injure." Nociceptors are commonly referred to as "pain receptors" because they initiate the electrical signals that reach the brain and elicit the unpleasant sensation of pain, but do not transmit "pain signals" themselves. The brain interprets nociceptive signals as pain. Nociceptors transmit signals that precede the subjective experience of pain.

Nociceptors are branched, free nerve endings that detect pain, pressure, and temperature. They respond to any stimulus that activates branches of the nerve ending itself, and, unlike other mechanoreceptors, are not associated with a single modality. They are most associated with painful stimuli. Free

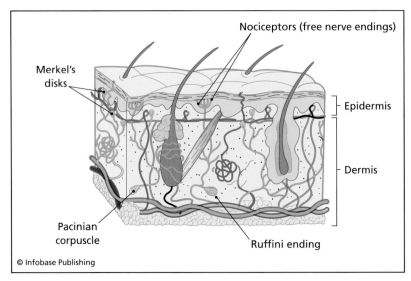

Figure 2.2 A number of different sensory receptors are found in the skin. Mechanoreceptors, such as Pacinian corpuscles, Ruffini endings, and Merkel's disks, respond to light touch and pressure. Nociceptors, or free nerve endings, sense painful stimuli that threaten to harm the body.

nerve endings are found throughout the skin in all regions of the body and are not connected to specialized receptor structures; however, they are surrounded by supportive cells called glia. They are associated with thinly or unmyelinated fibers grouped in bundles of the most superficial region of the dermis. **Myelin** is a protective fatty coat that surrounds and insulates axons.

Nociceptors can be categorized in a number of ways, depending on whether they are classified by the properties of their axons, or by what stimulus they best respond to. In terms of the size of the afferent fibers that innervate them and the types of stimuli they best respond to, nociceptors are classified as Aδ mechanical and C-polymodal groups. Both types are slowly adapting and have long-lasting activity, and it is thought that Aδ and C nociceptors mediate "first" and "second" pain, respectively; namely, the rapid, acute, sharp pain and, on the other hand, the delayed, more diffuse, dull pain caused by noxious stimuli. This is likely due to mechanisms of sensory-to-electrical signal conversion by the receptor, and/or the rate of conduction of their corresponding axon fibers.

Aδ mechanical nociceptors respond best to strong pressure and mechanical stimuli that cause damage to the skin. Mechanical nociceptors do not respond to noxious heat, cold, or irritant chemicals, but are selective for objects that produce pain. Typically they require relatively strong inputs to become activated, unlike Aβ receptors that receive information about non-painful stimuli, and for this reason are sometimes referred to as "high threshold mechanoreceptors." The receptive field of a mechanical nociceptor is large, covering up to 2 cm^2, and is made up of multiple nonoverlapping points. The axon that emerges from mechanical nociceptors is an **Aδ fiber.** The perceived quality of pain mediated by mechanical nociceptors is sharp, localized, prickling pain. Examples of stimuli that would activate Aδ receptors and fibers include cutting of the skin, strong blows to the body, and shearing forces on the skin.

C-polymodal nociceptors respond best to strong pressure, noxious heat and intense cold, and irritant chemicals (such as capsaicin, the "hot" component in chili peppers). C-polymodal nociceptors sense the temperature of the skin, and temperatures above 45°C (113°F), or below 27°C (81°F), a temperature that is colder than our body temperature of 37°C [98.6°F]), will activate them. The receptive field of C-polymodal nociceptors is one small non-overlapping region, with a density of 8 receptors per mm^2. The C-polymodal is the most numerous of both subclasses of nociceptors. **C-fibers** are associated with these nociceptors, which have a different function than Aδ mechanical receptors in that they signal a more long-term, dull, diffuse pain rather than a short-lived one. It is thought that this serves to tell the body not to overuse the damaged area.

CHEMORECEPTORS

In addition to responding to noxious sensory stimuli, sensory receptors called **chemoreceptors** are sensitive to a variety of chemicals, such as ions and molecules, that are locally released after injury to the skin and activate the chemoreceptors. Chemoreceptors at the site of injury detect this damage through a number of substances. These include (1) potassium, which is released by cells that have been damaged and whose contents leak out; (2) **serotonin**, which is released by blood cells called platelets that have been liberated due to cutting open a blood vessel in the skin; (3) bradykinin, which is also found in blood; (4) histamine, which is produced by immune cells called mast cells that are recruited to the area of tissue damage; (5) **prostaglandins**, which are created from a molecule called arachidonic acid that comes from the cell membranes of damaged cells; and (6) **substance P**, which is released by the incoming nerve fibers.

SENSORY TRANSDUCTION AND SIGNAL ENCODING

Once the peripheral receptors receive a sufficient activating stimulus, they convert this sensory energy into the electrical energy of a neural signal through transduction. For example, if an object exerts a strong enough amount of pressure on the skin, it will stretch the skin and deform the membrane of a Pacinian corpuscle that contains sodium channels. The inner pores of sodium channels will then stretch open, allowing sodium ions to rush through the membrane and into the corpuscle, causing a membrane depolarization and a small action potential to fire at the level of the receptor. This is called a **generator potential**, and it is not transmitted down the axon. When no physical contact is required to activate the nociceptors, such as in the case of C-polymodal nociceptors, generator potentials are created by less well understood mechanisms.

When the generator potential is large enough, a full action potential discharge is triggered in the initial segment of the axon, which travels the length of the sensory axon (Aβ, Aδ, C, etc.) to the neuron's cell body within the dorsal root ganglion. The **dorsal root ganglion (DRG)** is where the cell bodies of peripheral nerves reside. One end of the DRG extends to the periphery and the other to the spinal cord.

Nociception is unique in the way that individual sensory neurons and receptors have the ability to detect a number of different types of stimuli, for example, hot or cold. This is in contrast to the mechanoreceptive senses, where receptor structures are more highly specialized. This differential relay of a variety of information about the stimulus relies on **signal encoding**, where the nature of the stimulus is communicated in the precise sequence of action potentials created. All information about a stimulus must be encoded into the simple firing pattern of a neuron.

Because the action potential itself cannot change its fundamental properties (think of it as an all or none response, encoding a single binary piece of information: YES or NO), the pattern of action potential firing activity is the key to signal encoding. The ways a neuron can encode information are through intensity coding, temporal coding, and spatial coding.

Intensity encoding is the way a neuron increases or decreases its firing rate as a function of the strength of a stimulus. Intensity encoding directly translates stimulus intensity into a certain frequency of action potentials. This is the simplest and most common way the nervous system encodes information. For example, if pressure on the skin is strong, action potentials will fire at a rapid rate, and frequency will be high. Conversely, light pressure produces a lower frequency discharge rate. In some cases receptors produce an **opponent code**, constant discharging that can be altered by another stimulus. In this way a single receptor can encode two different types of stimuli by either increasing or decreasing the firing rate to one of two stimuli. For example, a thermoreceptor might produce a discharge of five spikes per second without stimulation, but in response to heat it would increase its firing rate to eight spikes per second, and for cold, decrease its firing rate to two spikes per second. Neurons in sensory pathways also vary in their sensitivity to a stimulus. Thus the proportion of cells activated by a stimulus also provides information about intensity.

The timing of action potential trains can relay information about the variation of stimulus strength over time, called **temporal coding**. Neurons may only fire at the onset and offset of stimulation, rather than firing throughout the duration of the application of the stimulus. This is a common characteristic of rapidly and slowly adapting neurons. Another example is the way a neuron would fire at the same time as a vibrating stimulus.

Spatial coding relays information concerning variations in stimulus strength over space in terms of which neurons are firing. This relies on neighboring receptive fields that project to neighboring regions of the **thalamus**, then cortex. The territories of receptive fields inform the brain about the physical extent of the stimulation.

■ **Learn more about the contents of this chapter** Search the Internet for *skin receptors*, *nociception*, and *Pacinian corpuscle.*

3 | The Viscera

As the skin acts as our sensory interface with the outside world, the viscera are our sensory interface with the internal world of our body. The insides of our hollow organs are effectively interacting with the external environment, within the confines of our body.

The viscera are made up of the soft internal organs of the body, particularly those contained within the abdominal and chest cavities (Figure 3.1). Visceral sensation serves more to alert the brain and body to damage to tissues rather than to more common types of sensation. We are not aware of feeling the muscular contractions of visceral organs, or their positions in the chest or abdomen, or how they are rubbing against each other, but we can certainly become aware of gas pains, kidney stones, heart attacks, and other painful visceral situations. Additionally, the possibility of interaction with potentially harmful food-borne agents necessitates protection by pain systems.

The mechanisms of visceral sensation and pain are quite different from those of the skin. Visceral pain has several distinct sensory characteristics and related mechanisms. One is that it is not evoked from all viscera; organs such as the liver, kidneys, lungs, and most solid viscera are not sensitive to painful stimuli. Some of these organs can be injured or damaged to a great degree without us feeling anything. For example, many diseases of the liver (cirrhosis caused by alcoholism) and lungs (emphysema due to smoking) are completely painless, and become noticed by the individual only because

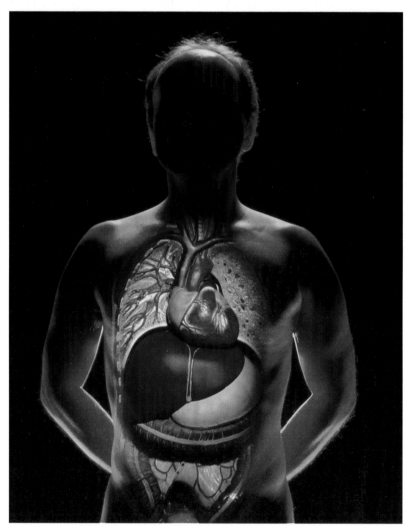

Figure 3.1 The human viscera are depicted in this model. The viscera include the heart, lung, kidneys, and the organs of the digestive and excretory systems.

the normal functioning of the organs becomes impaired, which produces other symptoms. On the other hand, relatively small injuries or damage to the stomach (such as by an ulcer), bladder (excessive fullness), or ureters (passing of a kidney stone) can cause severe pain. Unlike with the skin, there is not much of a relationship between the degree of tissue damage and the amount of pain, because not all visceral tissues are innervated by sensory receptors.

Second, visceral pain is not always directly linked to injury. For example, a car accident that traumatically tears the intestine causes no pain, whereas stretching of the bladder is painful. In these cases, the organs undergoing damage simply lack the receptors needed to translate damage into signals that would be perceived by the brain as painful.

Third, visceral pain is spread over a relatively large area. That is, if only a small portion of the viscera is experiencing some type of stimulation that causes pain, it is hard to precisely determine this location. This is due to the anatomical makeup of the visceral sensory system. Because there are very few visceral receptors, the sensory fibers are carried by a relatively smaller number of relay cells, and localizing pain to specific sites is difficult.

Fourth, visceral pain is referred to other locations of the body. This is due to the fact that visceral and skin sensory information converges on common relay pathways in the spinal cord, where mixing of signals occurs.

Finally, visceral pain is accompanied by motor and autonomic reflexes such as nausea, vomiting, and muscle tension, which serve to warn the body of impending danger, as well as to amplify this message.

RECEPTORS

The detection of visceral pain starts with sensory receptors located within the abdominal and thoracic cavities of the body.

Receptors are located in the mucosal linings of hollow visceral organs (such as the stomach, intestine, and colon); in membranes such as the peritoneum that surround the abdominal cavity and cover most of the abdominal organs; in the mesentery, a structure that attaches to the back wall of the abdominal cavity and supports the small intestines; and as individually distributed receptors involved in the regulation of secretion, movement of food through the intestine, and blood flow to the internal organs.

As with skin receptors, visceral receptors are generally classified by their responsiveness, and divided into two types: mechanoreceptors and nociceptors. But in contrast to the skin, where receptor densities are high, the viscera are only lightly innervated. Visceral receptors are found in very low density, with millimeters to centimeters between individual receptors, representing only about 5 percent of the density of skin afferent nerves leading from the skin to the central nervous system.

As with Pacinian corpuscles, visceral mechanoreceptors respond primarily to physical deformation of the receptor itself. They are found in the mesentery and in connective tissue around the viscera, as well as in the surface that surrounds the gut, heart, and lungs, and along blood vessels. The principal mechanical deformation that activates the receptors is stretching or swelling, called **distension**, from the internal pressure of hollow organs. This can be caused by rapid enlargement of the viscus by intestinal obstruction, forceful muscular contraction caused by passage of a kidney stone that causes a spasm of the muscular walls of structures carrying the stone as well as a buildup of fluids, and by rapid stretching of organs caused by the backup of fluids or gas. Other causes include compression of organs, ischemia (lack of oxygen), and interruption of blood flow, inflammation, muscle spasm, and traction.

Two distinct populations of visceral mechanoreceptors exist: a larger group (70–80 percent of total receptors) that has low thresholds for activation, and a smaller group (20–30 percent) that has high thresholds for response. Low-threshold receptors respond to stimuli within the normal physiologic range. For example, a large meal that causes stretching of the stomach would activate low-threshold receptors. High-threshold receptors respond preferentially to distending pressure that is likely to cause damage. For both, the firing rate encodes the magnitude of the stimulation.

Visceral nociceptors are found in the gastrointestinal tract, reproductive organs, and heart. Within the gut, they have multiple spot-like receptive fields in the gut lining. They do not respond to cutting, tearing, or crushing of the viscera, but they do respond to temperature and irritant chemical stimuli, especially to the products of inflammatory response, like their cor-

Visceral Sensitization

An interesting aspect of visceral pain is the potential for the development of increased sensitivity to stimulation following an injury or inflammation of an internal organ, called visceral hyperalgesia. For example, while an upset stomach or indigestion can cause pain in the organs directly affected, it can also cause pain in organs that are seemingly not affected, such as the bladder or gut. In these organs, normal functions such as urination or the movement of food through the intestine can become very painful. The mechanisms underlying visceral hyperalgesia are thought to be a change in the responsiveness of sensory neurons in the viscera such that they respond more intensely to naturally occurring stimuli.

responding skin nociceptors and chemoreceptors. Some visceral nociceptors become activated only after inflammation of their target organs.

TRANSMISSION

The viscera have dual sensory output pathways, with the majority of afferent fibers projecting to the spinal cord, and a smaller number of fibers projecting to the brain stem. The cell bodies of visceral afferent neurons destined for the spinal cord, in common with the cell bodies of skin afferent neurons, are located in dorsal root ganglia. But instead of passing only into the dorsal root ganglion and then the spinal cord, visceral afferents pass through or near structures called prevertebral ganglia and paravertebral ganglia. As a result, they are able to influence ganglion cell bodies that control the automatic features of the viscera involved in digestion and movement of food.

The number of spinal visceral afferent fibers is estimated to be less than 10 percent of the total spinal afferent input from all sources, including the skin. However, some compensation for the small number of visceral inputs is provided by the greater spread of afferent fiber inputs up and down the length of the cord. And individually, visceral afferent fibers possess more connections between neurons, called synapses, and enter the spinal cord at more locations than do skin afferents.

Visceral sensory axons are structurally and functionally the same as skin axons. From the skin, three major types of axons exist: large myelinated **Aβ fibers**, small myelinated Aδ fibers, and unmyelinated C-fibers. In visceral nerves, there are very few large myelinated Aβ fibers. Of the Aβ fibers that are present, they innervate Pacinian corpuscles located mostly in the mesenteries. The majority of afferent fibers are Aδ and C-fibers. The ratio of unmyelinated/myelinated fibers is about 10:1, which is quite the opposite of the ratio of skin fibers. This ratio suggests that both painful and non-painful information is carried by small Aβ and C-fibers.

Visceral afferents project into different segments of the spinal cord, depending on the location of the tissue or organ. Within the spinal cord, afferents terminate in superficial layers (**laminae**) I, II, and V. These are primarily thought to be pain-processing laminae. Visceral afferent fibers also terminate in lamina X, which surrounds the central part of the spinal cord called the central canal.

Once in the spinal cord, visceral information may be processed to some degree before it is sent upward by the spinal cord toward the brain. The major ascending spinal pathways involved in transmitting visceral information are the **spino-thalamic tract** and the dorsal column system. However, minor pathways convey information to the hypothalamus and reticular activating system.

BIOCHEMISTRY

Unlike skin afferent fibers that use both small and large neurotransmitter molecules for communication between afferents and second order spinal cord neurons, visceral afferent fibers primarily use large molecule peptides for signaling called **neuropeptides**. Neuropeptide transmitters have a much longer signaling effect (on the order of minutes to hours) than small molecule neurotransmitters. Neuropeptides found in visceral afferents are the same as those found in skin afferents, namely substance P and **calcitonin gene–related peptide (CGRP)**. In addition to peptides, however, serotonin is involved in visceral pain signaling.

Substance P is involved in both enhancing and inhibiting nociceptive signaling, depending on which receptor subtypes it activates, and in what part of the viscera. CGRP and serotonin are both important in sensitizing visceral afferent nerves.

■ **Learn more about the contents of this chapter** Search the Internet for *visceral pain*, *dorsal root ganglion*, and *neuropeptides*.

4 The Peripheral Nerve and Dorsal Root Ganglia

Within the somatosensory pathway between the skin (and also the viscera) and the spinal cord are the **primary afferent neurons**. The primary afferent neuron receives information from sensory receptors and transmits this information centrally to the spinal cord. From the outside inward, this primary afferent neuron can be divided into the peripheral nerve process, cell body, and central process. The peripheral nerve process receives input from the sensory receptor at its ending. The nerve consists of myelinated and unmyelinated axons that travel from the end process (sensory receptors) to the cell body (dorsal root ganglion), and away from the cell body into the spinal cord.

PERIPHERAL NERVE

The sensing end of the peripheral nerve receives information directly from sensory receptors in the skin or viscera and relays it to the cell body of the peripheral nerve through an axon. Just as not all sensory receptors are alike, neither are sensory axons. Sensory axons are classified primarily based on their diameter and whether they possess a myelin sheath.

Myelin is a fatty sheath that coats the axons of some neurons and serves to permit the efficient conduction of nerve impulses (Figure 4.1). Similar to the plastic insulation that surrounds electrical wires, myelin prevents current leakage by providing a high resistance barrier on the outside of nerves. Myelin is produced by cells called **oligodendrocytes** in the central nervous system, and by Schwann cells in the peripheral nervous system.

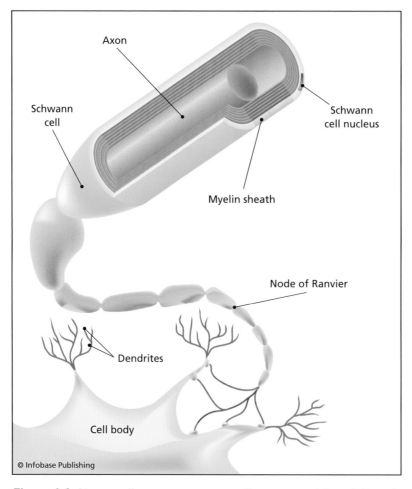

Axon

Schwann cell

Schwann cell nucleus

Myelin sheath

Node of Ranvier

Dendrites

Cell body

© Infobase Publishing

Figure 4.1 Nerve cells, or neurons, are often wrapped in a fatty substance known as myelin to increase the speed of transmission of nerve impulses. Within the nerve cell, the impulse travels down the axon where it is received by the dendrites of the cell body of an adjacent nerve cell.

Schwann cells form the myelin sheath around each axon, and are lined up in series along axons. Each Schwann cell wraps only a certain length of axon. Certain axons possess multiple thick wrappings by a single Schwann cell, effectively insulating it to a higher degree and allowing the axon to conduct its action potentials at a much higher velocity. The breaks in myelin between Schwann cell wrappings are called **nodes of Ranvier**, and these are the locations where action potentials are boosted along.

Conduction is the act of propagating action potentials along the length of an axon. While action potentials are smoothly conducted in unmyelinated axons, action potentials are conducted along myelinated axons between the nodes of Ranvier. This is termed **saltatory conduction**, from the Latin root *saltare*, meaning "to jump." Saltatory conduction utilizes node-to-node conduction of action potentials.

Axon fibers are subdivided by their degree of myelination. Large myelinated fibers termed **Aα fibers** are 13–20 micrometers in diameter. These fibers receive input from receptors in skeletal muscle and provide information to the nervous system regarding muscle position (**proprioception**). Medium-diameter myelinated fibers known as Aβ fibers are 6–12 micrometers in diameter, and transmit information received from mechanoreceptors. Small-diameter, thinly myelinated fibers termed Aδ fibers are 1–5 micrometers in diameter, and transmit information from the nociceptors about painful stimuli. Very thin unmyelinated fibers called C-fibers are 0.2–1.5 micrometers in diameter, and transmit information from nociceptors. Because of their differential myelin thickness, these axons all have conduction velocities that vary (Figure 4.2). Aβ fibers conduct impulses at a speed of 35–75 meters per second, smaller Aδ fibers conduct at 5–30 meters per second, and the finest C-fibers conduct impulses at 0.5–2 meters per second.

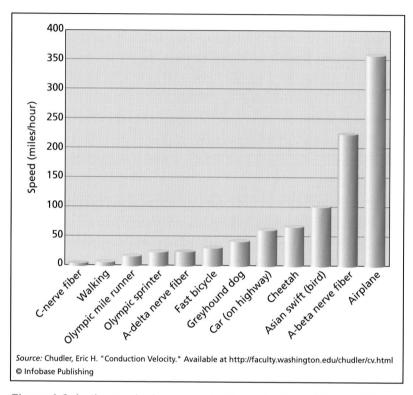

Source: Chudler, Eric H. "Conduction Velocity." Available at http://faculty.washington.edu/chudler/cv.html
© Infobase Publishing

Figure 4.2 In the graph above, conduction velocities of three different nerve fibers (purple) are compared to the speeds of various animals and modes of human transportation (green).

The Aδ and C-fibers can be thought of as pain-specific fibers because they are the fiber types primarily responsible for transmitting information from nociceptors. Aδ fibers are activated very rapidly and are associated with acute pain. These are considered "good pain" fibers because they warn the body about impending danger. C-fibers are activated more slowly, and are associated with diffuse, dull pain that is sometimes considered "bad pain" because it cannot be alleviated by removing the stimulus. An example of pain mediated by C-fibers is pain resulting from tissue damage.

Peripheral nerve axons are organized by **dermatomes**, regions of the body that are innervated by sensory fibers from a single spinal nerve. Going backward, the pathways of peripheral sensory nerves entering the spinal cord can be mapped to particular regions of the skin. Generally, these regions correspond to segments of the spinal cord where the nerves terminate. Innervation is overlapping to some degree so that damage to one spinal nerve does not necessarily result in complete lack of sensation in a corresponding skin zone. On a dermatome map, dermatomes appear to wrap the body like rings, except for the legs, where the dermatomes run the length of the legs.

The brain ultimately receives nerve impulses from specific dermatomes, whose location on the skin is determined by the specific axon carrying the message. This explains how the brain knows that a stimulus is occurring on the face rather than the

Shingles

Shingles is a disease that is characterized by an outbreak of rash or blisters on the skin. The symptoms of shingles often include burning or tingling pain, or sometimes numbness, in or under the skin. The virus that causes shingles is the same one that causes chicken pox—the varicella-zoster virus. Scientists think that during chicken pox, some of the virus particles leave the skin blisters and move into the dorsal root ganglion cell bodies of peripheral nerves that reside just outside the spinal cord, where they lie dormant. When the varicella-zoster virus reactivates, the virus moves back down the long nerve fibers that extend from the sensory cell bodies to the skin and cause the characteristic blisters of shingles in dermatome-specific patterns.

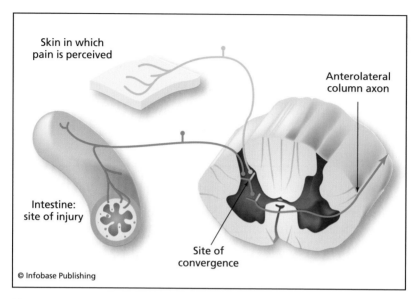

Skin in which
pain is perceived

Anterolateral
column axon

Intestine:
site of injury

Site of
convergence

© Infobase Publishing

Figure 4.3 Nerves from the skin and viscera often converge onto a single neuron in the dorsal horn of the spinal cord. Because of this, damage to the viscera (such as the intestine) may result in the sensation of pain on the skin near the organ. This phenomenon is known as referred pain.

arm, and makes it possible for the brain to keep track of which axon, or "line," the stimulus arrives on. Interestingly, internal organs do not posses direct axons/lines to the brain, so when there is damage to the organ, pain is experienced as **referred pain** on the skin near the organ. Referred pain is perceived in one area of the body when another (internal) area is actually receiving the painful stimulus (Figure 4.3). It is apparently caused by visceral (internal) and somatic (skin) nerves that synapse onto a common spinal cord projection neuron that ascends to the brain. Examples of referred pain include heart attack pain that manifests as pain that is felt in the left chest, shoulder, or jaw, and appendix pain that is experienced as pain in the umbilicus (belly button).

DORSAL ROOT GANGLION CELL BODY

The dorsal root ganglion (DRG) is a nodule on the peripheral nerve entering the spinal cord that contains cell bodies of afferent spinal nerve neurons (Figure 4.4). DRG neurons are among the physically longest cells in the body. Residing just outside the spinal cord, their peripheral projections must extend all the way to the skin of the arms and legs, a potential distance of several feet in humans. The DRG must be quite robust in order to manufacture all of the biochemicals needed for structural maintenance and functional operation at the cell body and synaptic locations. DRG neurons are unipolar neurons because they have a common input/output stalk that, at one end, is the peripheral process that receives information from sensory receptors, and has a central process that transmits this information centrally.

DRG neurons are most commonly classified by size, either large or small. A DRG's size correlates with the conduction velocity of its axon, and this conduction velocity is correlated with myelination, which, in turn, correlates with the type of information the axon is carrying. Small-diameter DRG neurons have small axons and are nociceptive, while large DRG neurons have large axons and are mechanoreceptive. DRG neurons are considered small if their diameter is less than 25 micrometers.

CENTRAL PROJECTION

Information is carried from the DRG cell body to the spinal cord through its central projection. From the perspective of the spinal cord, these are called spinal afferents. Depending on the type of sensory information being carried, DRG neurons send their spinal projections into the spinal cord, where they either project upward toward the brain, or into the spinal cord gray matter, where they make synaptic connections.

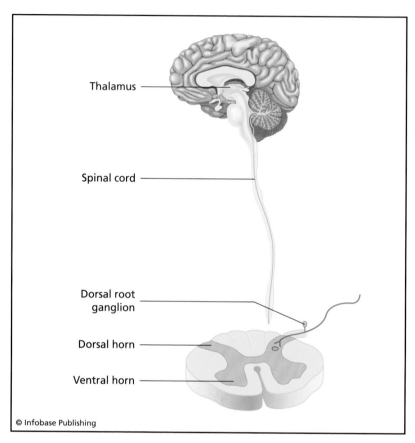

Thalamus

Spinal cord

Dorsal root
ganglion

Dorsal horn

Ventral horn

Figure 4.4 The dorsal root ganglion contains cell bodies of spinal neurons that connect the body and spinal cord. The axons of these neurons innervate many parts of the body, including muscle, skin, bone, and the visceral organs.

Aβ afferents enter the spinal cord and can either ascend toward the brain, or synapse first. C-fibers make their primary synaptic terminations in lamina II, also known as the substantia gelatinosa, which is a major pain-specific relay region of the spinal cord. C-fibers also synapse on neurons in laminae III–VI. Central projections of DRG neurons utilize a number of small-molecule and peptide neurotransmitters in their communication with second-order neurons in the pathway.

■ **Learn more about the contents of this chapter** Search the Internet for *Schwann cell*, *myelin sheath*, and *nerve impulse*.

5 | The Spinal Cord

The spinal cord is primarily a carrier of information, but it also performs a large degree of information processing. It receives information from the skin, muscles, and internal organs, and transfers signals upward toward the brain. The spinal cord was once thought to act only as a channel of information transfer between the body and the brain, but now we know that the spinal cord plays a key role not only in transferring, but also in processing pain and sensory information.

ANATOMY OF THE SPINAL CORD

The spinal cord extends from the base of the skull down to the lower back, and is a continuous structure that is not anatomically interrupted. The spinal cord is protected by a bony structure called the vertebral column, sometimes referred to as the backbone. The vertebral column acts as a hard casing to prevent the spinal cord from being damaged by external forces. In humans, the vertebral column is made up of individual **vertebrae** that are stacked up and surround the spinal cord in rings. The vertebrae are connected to each other by ligaments that are flexible enough to allow the back to bend.

Contained within the smooth inner walls of the vertebral column is the spinal cord itself. The outside of the spinal cord is wrapped in a sheath of membranes called the **meninges**. The first such layer is called the **dura mater** (Latin for "tough mother"). The dura mater is a tough fibrous casing that acts both as a physical and biochemical barrier. The dura mater is exquisitely resistant to tearing or being broken open by physical forces. Along with blood vessels, it is also a principal component of the blood-brain barrier, a system that acts as a barrier to infection and toxic substances. The **blood-brain barrier** is not a physical barrier, however, and it does allow the selective passage of nutrients, oxygen-carrying blood cells, and other vital substances into the spinal cord. Blood that is purified by this barrier becomes a clear liquid called **cerebrospinal fluid** that surrounds the spinal cord, bathing it in nutrients. The spinal cord has roughly the same density as cerebrospinal fluid and thus is buoyant in it, partly because of a ribbon-like ligament that runs along both sides of the cord and suspends it inside the protective surrounding dural sheath, where spinal nerves travel. The space is also referred to as the **intrathecal space**. The **epidural space** is located outside the dural sheath. During childbirth, pain-reducing drugs are often administered directly into the epidural space through a needle, effectively blocking all pain signals originating from the uterus from reaching the spinal cord.

Both the vertebrae and spinal cord are divided into distinct regions (Figure 5.1): The cervical curvature runs from the base of the skull to the lower neck and is comprised of seven vertebrae (C1–C7), the thoracic curvature runs from the shoulders down to the lower body and is made up of twelve vertebrae (T1–T12), and the lumbar curvature is made up of five vertebrae (L1–L5) and extends down to the sacrum, in the middle of the pelvis. The **cauda equina** is the remaining bundle of nerve axons that travel out of the cord to the lower body. The spinal cord proper ends at L1, and terminates in a pointed end called the **conus medullaris**. A strand of connective tissue that contains nerve roots, called the **filum terminale**, extends through the conus and attaches to the cocygeal vertebra at the bottom of the spinal column.

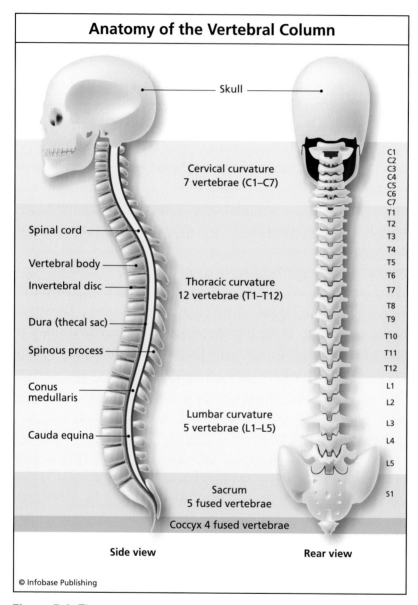

Anatomy of the Vertebral Column

Skull

Cervical curvature
7 vertebrae (C1–C7)

C1
C2
C3
C4
C5
C6
C7
T1
T2
T3
T4
T5
T6
T7
T8
T9
T10
T11
T12
L1
L2
L3
L4
L5
S1

Spinal cord

Vertebral body

Invertebral disc

Dura (thecal sac)

Spinous process

Conus
medullaris

Cauda equina

Thoracic curvature
12 vertebrae (T1–T12)

Lumbar curvature
5 vertebrae (L1–L5)

Sacrum
5 fused vertebrae

Coccyx 4 fused vertebrae

Side view

Rear view

© Infobase Publishing

Figure 5.1 The vertebral column consists of 24 individual vertebrae that are divided into the cervical, thoracic, and lumbar regions. At the bottom of the column are two sections of fused vertebrae: the sacrum and coccyx.

The cervical and lumbar sections of the spinal cord are distinctly thicker in diameter than the thoracic segments due to their unique roles in sending and receiving motor and sensory commands to large areas of the body—the arms and legs. All input and output to and from the arms is carried through the lower cervical segments. All input and output to and from the legs is similarly carried through the lumbar enlargement. Because there are more nerve fibers traveling in and out of the spinal cord at these locations, the cord is correspondingly larger in diameter in these spots, which are known as the **cervical enlargement** (C3–T1) and the **lumbar enlargement** (L1–S3), respectively.

The nerves that enter and exit the spinal cord are called **spinal nerves**, and can be divided into sensory or motor nerves. The sensory nerves carry information into the spinal cord from the skin or body and enter into the spinal cord at the dorsal surface. Motor nerves exit the spinal cord through the **ventral** surface and make their way out to muscles. In humans, there are 31 pairs of spinal nerves: 8 cervical, 12 thoracic, 5 lumbar, 5 sacral, and 1 coccygeal. Several spinal nerves often join together in interconnected fibers called a **plexus** that forms a peripheral nerve. An example of a plexus that originates from the cervical enlargement is the brachial plexus. It contains various nerves of the arm, including the median nerve, which connects to the top part of the arm and elbow, wrist, and fingers.

Cut in cross (transverse) section, like a piece of bread from a loaf, the spinal cord is divided into areas of lighter colored tissue called **white matter**, and darker regions called **gray matter**. White matter surrounds the inner butterfly-shaped gray matter (Figure 5.2). Each of these 2 major regions of the cord has a different role. The white matter is comprised mainly of nerve fibers traveling up or down the cord, carrying signals from the

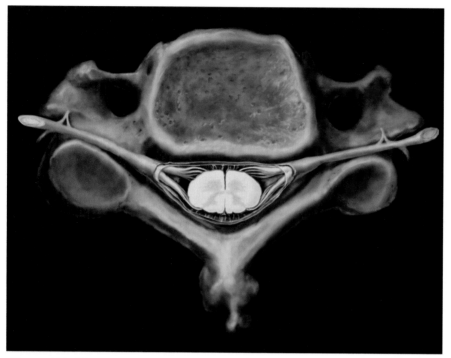

Figure 5.2 The spinal cord is visible in the center of this illustration of a cervical vertebra. The butterfly-shaped portion of the spinal cord is the gray matter, which is surrounded by the white matter.

body to the brain, or in the opposite direction from the brain to the body carrying motor commands. The white matter can be thought of as the highway system of the spinal cord, where information is communicated up and down in high-speed lines. Gray matter is the portion of the spinal cord where incoming afferent signals are received from the periphery, processed to some degree, and routed into the white matter up toward the brain. The white matter is also the location where descending white matter pathways make connections onto spinal output neurons, sending **efferent** commands out to the muscles.

The white matter carries information up and down the spinal cord in specific fiber bundles called **tracts,** located in distinct anatomical regions. The dorsal funiculus (the anatomical area of the spinal cord that is located near the top, in the middle) carries information to the brain from the body regarding light touch, brush, vibration, and related stimuli. This region is known as the **dorsal column system**. In the lateral portion of the spinal cord are various other tracts that travel up or down the length of the cord. The ventrolateral quadrant of the cord carries the spinothalamic tract, which carries information from the body to the brain regarding temperature and painful stimuli. Descending tracts that influence the pain system, such as the **raphaespinal tract**, which sends pain-dampening commands from a collection of nuclei called the **raphe nuclei** to the gray matter, are also located in this region.

The gray matter can be divided functionally into two major components: the **dorsal horn** and the **ventral horn** (see Figure 4.4). The dorsal horn is the portion of gray matter that deals mainly with sensory processing. Incoming afferent fibers from the dorsal root ganglion (DRG) synapse here onto dorsal horn neurons that are the cells of origin of the spinothalamic tract. **Primary afferent fibers** are both functionally and anatomically divided based on their sensory modality, speed of transmission, and thickness.

Two major types of neurons are located in the dorsal horn: cell bodies of tract/projection neurons, and **interneurons**. Interneurons are the cells that receive afferent inputs and do the majority of processing before relaying information over a short distance to the cell bodies of tracts that make up the starting point of ascending sensory tracts. Neurons and supporting cells are localized to anatomical layers called laminae. Certain laminae, such as laminae I through IV, are associated with specific functions such as receiving sensory input, processing this input, and relaying it to white matter tracts such as the spinothalamic and dorsal column system. The most superficial, lamina I, almost exclusively receives inputs from Aδ fibers, whereas laminae II–VI receive inputs from all fiber types.

Dorsal horn output neurons, if relaying information exclusively about pain, temperature, and crude touch, send their axons along the spinothalamic tract, located near the periphery of the spinal cord. Emerging fibers first cross over to the opposite ("contralateral") side of the cord through lamina X in the ventral white crossing-over area before ascending.

From the spinal cord, axons ascend upward to the brain and make primary connections in the thalamus, a major relay and integration site, located deep in the core of the brain. The thalamus then sends pain signals upward to the cerebral **cortex**, the outermost surface of the brain where neural impulses are finally interpreted as complex sensations that we are aware of and experience.

The ventral horn is made up of large output neurons called α- and γ-motor neurons. These relay motor commands from the descending motor pathways to skeletal muscles. Commands to the heart, diaphragm, and internal organs such as the stomach are communicated in a different system. Although little information processing takes place in this region, pain reflex pathways use these neurons to rapidly perform motor actions without communicating with the brain directly.

PHYSIOLOGY AND BIOCHEMISTRY

Primary afferent fibers from the DRG enter the spinal cord and synapse on one or multiple cells in the dorsal horn. Different **neurotransmitter** molecules communicate between different afferent fiber types and second-order cells. Neurotransmitters are synthesized in the presynaptic neurons and are released by the terminal endings of these neurons. They move across the gap between neurons, known as the synaptic cleft, and bind to receptors on the terminals of post-synaptic neurons.

Afferent fibers utilize a few common neurotransmitters. Neurotransmitters have either excitatory or inhibitory effects on the firing probability of post-synaptic neurons. These include the excitatory amino acid neurotransmitter **glutamate**, which is the most abundant neurotransmitter substance involved in nerve signaling. A subclass of glutamate receptors known as **NMDA** receptors are found on post-synaptic neurons of the dorsal horn, in pain-processing laminae. **ATP** also excites neurons in superficial laminae that process mechanical and/or painful inputs, but it is thought that its role is less pain-specific.

Neuropeptides, signaling molecules somewhat larger than neurotransmitters, also participate in pain signaling between neurons. Neuropeptides are released in smaller quantities, but due to their complexity they exert a more pronounced effect on the post-synaptic neuron. Two such molecules found in the terminals of small-diameter afferent fibers are substance P and calcitonin–gene related peptide. Substance P is located almost exclusively in pain-carrying small-diameter unmyelinated afferent fibers that synapse in high degree in superficial layers of the dorsal horn. Its name comes from early experiments where it was implicated in pain processing, i.e., "substance pain." Substance P is released by these fibers following painful mechanical, thermal, or chemical stimulation of the skin. Substance P is also found in neurons intrinsic to the spinal dorsal horn. Preferentially binding substance P receptors are found within corresponding pain-processing laminae I and II.

Calcitonin–gene related peptide (CGRP) is often found within the same presynaptic storage vesicles as substance P. CGRP is found in small thinly myelinated and unmyelinated afferents which possess terminals in laminae I–II and V. CGRP binding sites correspond to pain-processing laminae, and include I–VI, some of which may or may not have a direct role in pain processing. Similar to substance P, noxious mechanical and thermal stimulation elicits the release of CGRP, which is thought to enhance the actions of substance P.

Inhibitory neurotransmitters associated with sensory and pain processing include **GABA** and glycine, the monoamines, and peptide molecules such as the opioids. GABA is found primarily in smaller neurons called interneurons that do not directly carry information from the periphery to the spinal cord, but instead participate in the relay and processing of sensory and painful stimuli between afferent fibers and output neurons of the spinothalamic tract. GABA is found in interneurons of the most superficial laminae of the cord, I–III. **Glycine** is found in neurons and presynaptic terminals in the superficial dorsal horn. Both GABA and glycine act presynaptically, such that they are able to prevent firing. GABA and glycine both also act directly on dorsal horn interneurons to inhibit their discharge activity. GABA exerts its effects by binding to two distinct receptors, $GABA_A$ and $GABA_B$. The $GABA_A$ receptors form a Cl⁻ ion channel, and binding of GABA to $GABA_A$ receptors increases the Cl⁻ flow (conductance) of presynaptic neurons, further increasing the polarity of the neuron.

Monoamines are a group of neurotransmitters that possess a modified amino acid, and include serotonin, norepinephrine, and acetylcholine. Monoamines are not produced in either primary afferent fibers or in dorsal horn neurons, but rather in the brain where projections are sent down to the spinal cord that synapse on sensory neurons. The overall effect of monoamines is to set the "tone" of the processing, i.e., to permit or dampen sensory transmission. Serotonin (also known as 5-HT, after its chemical formula), can be found in the presynaptic terminals of descending raphaespinal fibers in the dorsal horn. The raphe nuclei are a cluster of serotonin-producing cells in the brain stem. Serotonin-containing fibers synapse on both interneurons and relay neurons of the cord, and in general, inhibit firing of these cells, reducing the transmission of pain information to the brain. **Norepinephrine** projections originate in a large nucleus within the brain stem called the locus coeruleus, and, like the raphaespinal fibers, descend down the length of the cord. Termination of these fibers occurs in the superficial laminae (I and II) as well as in deeper laminae associated with output (IV–VI). Stimulation of the locus coeruleus causes release of norepinephrine in the spinal cord, which results in inhibition of dorsal horn pain neurons through hyperpolarization (in a manner similar to GABA, but with another ion, K^+), typically excited by glutamate.

Neuropeptides with an overall inhibitory effect on pain neurons are classified a number of different ways. The most prevalent and potent inhibitory peptides are the opioids. **Opioids** were named as such because naturally occurring substances in the seeds of the opium poppy plant were found to activate this system experimentally. The anti-pain medication morphine acts on the opioid system. Opioid peptides are present in interneurons and synaptic terminals. Opiate receptors are found in high amounts in the superficial dorsal horn on both presynaptic and post-synaptic neurons. The release of opioids is under partial control of descending fibers from the brain. The overall effects of the opioids are to depress the responses of dorsal horn neurons. Additionally, the excitatory responses of dorsal horn neurons evoked by excitatory amino acids are inhibited by opioids.

CONTROL AND PROCESSING

The control of the processing of incoming sensory and pain signals by dorsal horn neurons is maintained by local and nonlocal elements. Intrinsic control is governed by interneurons, which make up small networks that modulate the excitability of major neurons. Extrinsic modulation is achieved through descending projections. This system of pathways originates in different regions of the brain whose axon fibers course down through the spinal cord to synapse, at all levels of the cord, on pain processing neurons such as raphaespinal and descending fibers carrying norepinephrine.

Some descending axons synapse and act directly on spinal neurons, while others synapse on spinal neurons indirectly through a number of linked neurons, or through small networks. In the case of a multisynaptic connection, the net outcome is likely to be inhibitory; however, activation of the network is itself excitatory. For example, the descending control axon might synapse on, and excite, an interneuron that has an inhibitory effect on its target output pain neuron, such that in this case the net effect is inhibition. This simple configuration allows not only a control of the final output neuron, but permits the integration of a number of simultaneously converging inputs by the interneurons, and eventual combined modulation of the output neuron.

Surprisingly, the spinal cord processes a significant amount of sensory and pain information before sending it upward toward the brain. This processing exists in the form of interneurons, convergent output neurons, and small local networks of neurons. In most cases, these elements assimilate the information relayed into them like small computers, integrating the type, intensity, rate, and other fundamental properties relating to the painful stimulus. In the simplest type of processing, these elements add, subtract, multiply, and divide incoming excitatory and inhibitory signals, and relay the "answer" to output cells. A good analogy of how these systems work is that of the chairperson of a meeting. In this case, the "decision" of the output cell is modulated by the single representative who takes into account the votes of all members.

OUTPUT

The dorsal column system is the main fiber tract by which the spinal cord sends information about fine touch and limb

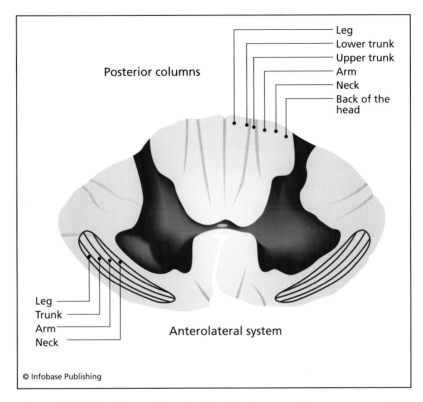

Leg
Lower trunk
Upper trunk
Arm
Neck
Back of the head

Posterior columns

Leg
Trunk
Arm
Neck

Anterolateral system

© Infobase Publishing

Figure 5.3 This illustration depicts the topographic arrangement of ascending tracts of the spinal cord. Axons relaying sensory information to the brain from the skin are arranged within discrete regions of the spinal cord white matter.

position in space (proprioception) to the brain. After Aβ afferents destined to travel in the dorsal column system have entered the spinal cord, they do not make any synaptic connections in the gray matter. This is in contrast to other fiber types that do terminate in the superficial dorsal horn. Instead, they enter the dorsal funiculus in the middle of the cord. Once in the dorsal funiculus, the Aβ axon courses upward toward the medulla, where it synapses on the same side at which it entered the cord. The medulla is the bottom part of the brain that makes up the brain stem, positioned between the spinal cord and brain. The ascending axon terminates in the medulla on the same side, in either the **nucleus gracilis** or **nucleus cuneatus**, then projects from one of these nuclei to the thalamus, and on to the sensory cortex for perception.

There are two major components that make up the dorsal column system, the **fasciculus gracilis**, and the **fasciculus cuneatus**. In Latin, the word *fasciculus* means "little bundle," and this is precisely what is found in the dorsal column system—little bundles of axons. *Gracilis* and *cuneatus* mean "slender," and "wedge," respectively. Depending on which level of the spinal cord the Aβ afferent enters from (i.e., the arms or the legs), it travels in either the fasciculus gracilis or fasciculus cuneatus. If the afferent enters from T6 and above, it travels in the fasciculus cuneatus. If the afferent enters from T7 and below, it travels in the fasciculus gracilis. Because the fasciculus gracilis contains fibers from spinal cord levels lower than fasciculus cuneatus, the fasciculus gracilis lies more toward the middle of the spinal cord than does the fasciculus cuneatus. In other words, fibers from the lower limbs project more medially, while fibers from the upper limbs project more laterally. This is because axons are added into the dorsal column system in an inside-out manner (Figure 5.3). Axons traveling in the fasciculus gracilis terminate in the nucleus gracilis, while fibers in fasciculus cuneatus synapse in the ipsilateral nucleus cuneatus.

From these nuclei, the dorsal column axons cross the midline of the brain stem and ascend through the medial lemniscus to synapse on neurons within the thalamus on the opposite side of the brain. Specifically, they synapse in the ventral posterior nucleus of the thalamus, and from there, neurons project to the primary sensory cortex.

The dorsal column system has traditionally been thought to relay information related only to fine touch and proprioception, but recently it has been shown to convey information about visceral pain. Experimental and clinical evidence indicates that sensory information from the viscera reaches the thalamus largely via a spinal cord pathway that originates from dorsal column neurons, ascends in the dorsal column, and relays in the fasciculus gracilis onto neurons that connect with the thalamus.

The conveyance of pain information from dorsal horn output cells is relatively simple. Small and large neurons in both superficial and deeper dorsal horn laminae send their axons up to the brain. While projections from spinal neurons can travel in many distinct pathways, the majority of pain-carrying fibers form the spinothalamic tract. These axons cross the spinal cord and ascend on the opposite side of the body. It is not known why this crossing-over occurs. The spinothalamic tract itself is located in the ventrolateral quadrant of the spinal cord white matter, near the ventral horn gray matter. It runs the length of the spinal cord and becomes thicker as more axons enter it higher along the spinal cord. Its termination is supraspinal, meaning "above the spinal cord," in the brain stem and thalamus.

Within the brain stem, the spinothalamic tract synapses on clusters of brain stem neurons within descending control nuclei, such as the raphe magnus and locus coeruleus. In the case of the raphe magnus, this connection from the spinothalamic tract serves to inform the raphe magnus that the spinal cord is receiving painful information that requires dampening. The nucleus raphe magnus in turn increases its inhibitory modulation of pain signals entering the spinal cord, effectively turning down the intensity of the painful stimulus.

The majority of spinothalamic fibers are directed toward the thalamus where they synapse on third-order neurons within specific thalamic nuclei. If neurons of the spinothalamic tract receive their primary inputs from receptive fields on the face, projections are made to the ventral posterior medial nucleus. This is located in the lower back middle portion of the thalamus. If the spinothalamic tract neurons possess receptive fields elsewhere on the body, projections terminate in the ventral posterior lateral nucleus. The medial thalamus and intralaminar nuclei of the thalamus also receive spinal inputs. From the thalamus, projections are sent to the cortex, where pain is interpreted. Supraspinal projections ultimately function to alert us to more sophisticated aspects of pain, and permit the development of memories associated with the pain and higher cognitive functions.

The second type of output is simpler. Rather than ascending toward the brain in the spinothalamic tract, the output of spinal neurons remains within the spinal cord and is sent directly to motor neurons of the ventral horn of the spinal cord. This primitive **reflex arc** pathway evolved very early as a way of protecting the body against potentially damaging events. This is a very short loop of axons that can react with very high speed; excitation of motor output cells drives muscular contraction in response to painful stimuli, and no supraspinal processing is required for this protective loop to be activated. The reflex arc consists of five major components: (1) the receptor at the end of the sensory neuron in the skin that detects a painful stimulus; (2) the sensory afferent neuron that enters the spinal cord and conveys the pain impulse to dorsal horn neurons; (3) integration components such as an interneuron or output cell that synapses onto a motor neuron; (4) the motor neuron efferent that conducts the nerve impulse out of the spinal cord down a peripheral nerve toward a target; and (5) that target itself, which is typically a muscle fiber group that contracts and moves the part of the body receiving the painful stimulus away from the source of the stimulus (Figure 5.4).

Spinal reflex arcs require a minimum of two neurons: a sensory neuron (input) and a motor neuron (output). The classic

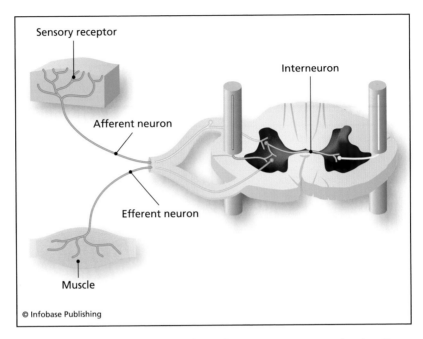

Figure 5.4 The reflex arc begins when a sensory receptor is stimulated. The afferent neuron then carries an impulse toward the spinal cord, where it contacts a neuron in the dorsal horn. The impulse is carried away from the spinal cord by an efferent neuron toward a muscle or other target.

example of such an arc is the "withdrawal reflex." In this case, the sensory neuron synapses directly onto a motor neuron, and when activated by a painful stimulus such as a hot stove, excites the motor neuron that activates the muscle necessary to withdraw the hand from the stove. **Polysynaptic** reflex arcs involve more than one synaptic connection. In most cases there is an interneuron that acts as an integrator and directs the pain impulse to a number of output neurons that control different muscle groups. Stepping on a tack, for example, not only activates the muscles in the affected leg to flex and pull away from the tack, but also activates the opposite leg to extend and move the rest of the body away from the painful stimulus.

Other muscle groups such as those in the arms and trunk can be innervated in polysynaptic reflex circuits to adjust and accommodate the changes in body position and posture associated with jumping backward, as well as to recruit the brain stem and thalamic nuclei to aid in dampening the pain signal.

■ **Learn more about the contents of this chapter** Search the Internet for *ventral horn, substance P, interneuron, synapse,* and *withdrawal reflex.*

6 | The Brain

Neither sensation nor pain exists until the brain becomes involved. That is to say, until sensory or nociceptive signals travel into the spinal cord, up and through the brain stem or thalamus, and reach the cortex, they are just that—sensory impulses. It is the higher-order processing of the cortex that interprets these impulses as sensory signals and applies these signals to our consciousness where the experience of the sensation originates. The brain receives incoming sensory signals and routes them to a number of different locations, each assigning a different interpretive meaning to the signals. In the case of pain, for example, the brain decides where the pain is taking place, the so-called sensory/discriminative aspect of pain, as well as what it feels like as an unpleasant sensation, the affective component of pain.

The route from the skin or visceral receptors to the cortex is called the sensory projection system. Each receptor in the skin has its own dedicated pathway to the cortex, through connections in the spinal cord or brain stem, and thalamus. Each has its own area of the cortex reserved for its processing.

THALAMUS
Before somatosensory signals reach the cortex, they must first pass through the thalamus, a gray matter relay center in the core of the brain (Figure 6.1). The thalamus is located

in the center of the brain, beneath the cerebral hemispheres and adjacent to the third ventricle. The primary role of the thalamus is to process and relay sensory information from most sensory pathways to the cerebral cortex. The thalamus receives information from nearly all sensory systems of the body, including touch, pain, vision, hearing, taste, and balance; the only exception is smell.

Remember that the spinal cord and brain stem are capable of making reflex decisions without signals passing through the thalamus and into the cortex for processing. The conscious perception of a stimulus, however, requires that a signal must be routed to the thalamus as well. An example of this is the reflex associated with touching a hot stove—the spinal reflex within

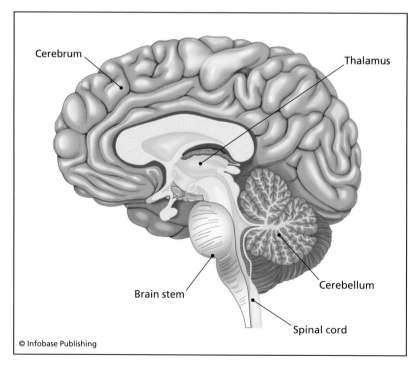

© Infobase Publishing

Figure 6.1 The thalamus serves as a processing and relay station for information to and from the cerebral cortex, also known as the cerebrum.

the spinal cord takes care of removing the hand from the stove, but a signal is simultaneously sent to the brain and informs us about what is happening.

Each ascending sensory pathway that originates in the spinal cord that is destined to reach the cortex, be it the spinothalamic tract or dorsal column system, converges in the thalamus. The region of the thalamus that receives sensory information is called the ventral posterior complex, given its anatomical location. (Although this is generally true, there are other areas of the thalamus that also receive sensory information, e.g., the medial thalamic nuclei.) This complex is made up of lateral and medial nuclei that receive inputs from different parts of the body. Located more toward the outside of the thalamus is the ventral posterior lateral (VPL) nucleus, which receives projections from the dorsal column medial lemniscus pathway and the spinothalamic tract, carrying all sensory and pain information from the body and back of the head. Located more toward the middle of the thalamus is the ventral posterior medial (VPM) nucleus, which receives axons from the trigeminal nerve, carrying information from the face regarding touch and pain signals. As all skin input from the entire body passes through the sensory relay of the ventral posterior complex of the thalamus, it contains a complete representation of the entire body.

Axons of VPL neurons project through the **internal capsule**, a thick bundle of axons that fan outward from the thalamus to the cerebral cortex. This thalamocortical pathway is often called the somatosensory radiation, and it is the major route by which the thalamus connects to the cerebral cortex. The shape of the entire fiber system of the internal capsule is like the bell of a trumpet. The posterior limb of the internal capsule carries fibers directly from the VPL and VPM nuclei to the sensory cortex.

The internal capsule fibers carrying sensory information terminate in a general region of the brain called the postcentral gyrus in the parietal lobe. The postcentral gyrus is a raised region

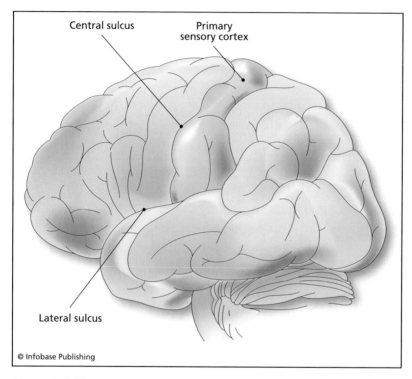

Figure 6.2 The primary sensory cortex processes information received from the skin, muscles, bones, tendons, and joints. It plays a role in the processing of pain.

located just behind a major groove in the brain called the central sulcus, and it wraps across the top surface of the brain in a left-right manner. It is the location of the **primary sensory cortex**, the main sensory receptive area for touch and pain (Figure 6.2).

Other nuclei of the thalamus that receive sensory information from the spinal cord are the ventral medial posterior nucleus (VMPo) and medial dorsal nucleus. The VMPo projects to the insular cortex and may be the key relay for pain signals to reach the **amygdala**, a major brain center related to the emotions. The medial dorsal nucleus also projects to the amygdala through a structure called the cingulated gyrus that is involved in emotion and memory.

CORTEX

The pattern of termination of sensory information is **somatotopic** in that its surface corresponds to a mapping of the surface shape of the body. There is a map of sensory space called a **homunculus**, Latin for "little man," in this location. For the primary sensory cortex, this is called the sensory homunculus (Figure 6.3). The homunculus is used to map out a human figure onto the primary sensory cortex that reflects the relative sensory space our body parts represent. The legs and trunk are represented on the middle surface of the primary sensory cortex, and the arms and hands on the outside surface. The face is represented near the bottom aspect. The homunculus does not represent the body surface in actual proportions. When neurosurgeons first mapped out the cortex by stimulating it electrically and having the patient report where they felt stimulation on their bodies, it was found that the mapped fields were exceptionally large for the lips, face, hands, and genitals. These parts of the body are considerably more sensitive than other parts of the body, so the homunculus has abnormally large lips, hands, and genitals. This is reflected anatomically by the greater number of neurons within these areas of the primary sensory cortex dedicated to processing sensory information from these skin areas.

Specifically within the primary sensory cortex, axons from the thalamus synapse on cortical neurons located primarily in layer IV of the somatic sensory cortex. This layer is the input layer of the cortex. Much like the superficial laminae of the spinal cord dorsal horn that receive sensory information from the skin or viscera, layer IV is the upstream recipient of this information. Interneurons in layer IV then feed information to other layers of the cortex that direct its output to other regions of the cortex or deeper brain structures.

The primary sensory cortex is made up of four distinct regions known as **Brodmann's areas** (areas 3a, 3b, 1, and 2). Regions are numbered given their location on the cortical

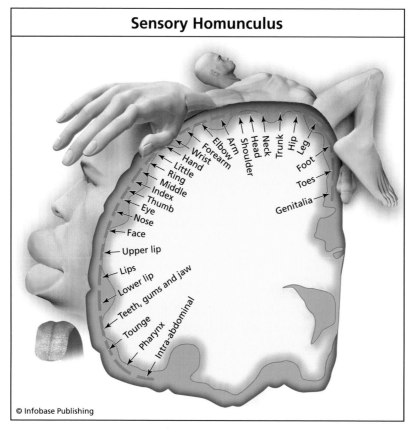

Figure 6.3 The small human figure shown here, called a homunculus, is commonly used to reflect the relative sensory or motor space our body parts occupy on the cerebral cortex.

map. Although area 3b is generally known as the primary sensory cortex, all four areas are involved in processing tactile information. Neurons in areas 3b and 1 process skin stimuli, neurons in 3a process stimuli related to proprioception, and area 2 neurons process both tactile and proprioceptive stimuli. These are areas of the cortex that are distinguished by differences in the arrangement and density of neurons in their six cellular layers and are identified by numbers. As a historical mapping system based on anatomy that has since been better characterized, the numbering system is still used to describe cortical locations that control different functions of the nervous system and the body.

HIGHER-ORDER PROCESSING

Although the primary sensory cortex is involved in the localization of pain on the body, other parts of the cortex are important in processing the motivational aspects of pain. The reception of pain signals by the secondary somatosensory and limbic cortex gives these messages an emotional and "feeling" dimension. Sensory information is distributed from the primary sensory cortex to these higher-order cortical and deeper brain structures.

The **secondary sensory cortex** receives connections from the adjacent primary sensory cortex, and sends projections deeper into the brain to structures of the **limbic system**, which is associated with the emotions. These include the amygdala and **hippocampus**, which are involved in emotion, and in learning and memory, respectively (Figure 6.4). The limbic system is responsible for producing an immediate emotional response to sensory stimulation. This sensory pathway is also important in forming long-lasting impressions, feelings, and memories associated with sensory experiences, and it is especially activated during extreme sensory experiences—either painful or pleasant.

The **parietal lobe** is a major lobe of the brain that incorporates the secondary sensory cortex. Its location is just behind the frontal cortex, and in front of the occipital cortex, in the rear of the brain. It lies just above the temporal lobe, on the sides of the brain. The primary functions of the parietal lobe are to integrate sensory information from various senses, and in the mental manipulation of objects. The occipital and temporal lobes receive visual and auditory signals, respectively. As a result of the location of the parietal cortex, encompassing loosely defined borders between these other lobes, it can receive combined inputs from them. As such, the parietal lobe plays an important role in integrating sensory information from various senses, and in the manipulation of objects. Portions of the

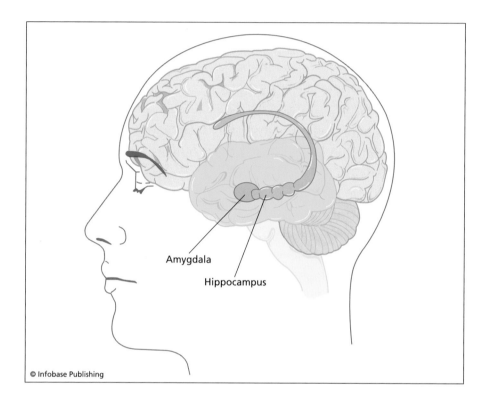

Figure 6.4 The amygdala and hippocampus are part of the brain's limbic system, which is involved in emotion, learning, and memory.

parietal lobe are involved with processing visual and spatial information. This area is known as the **parietal association area**. Much less is known about this lobe than others, probably because its functions are quite sophisticated.

The parietal lobes can be divided into two main functional regions. The first involves sensation and perception, while the other is involved with integrating sensory input, primarily from the visual system. The first region integrates the multiple forms of sensory and/or painful information to form a single perception, or cognition. The second region constructs a spatial coordinate system to represent the world around us in a three-dimensional space within the brain. This portion of the parietal cortex helps us to localize pain to a particular region of the body in space. Individuals with damage to the parietal lobes often show striking and surprising deficits, such as abnormalities in sensing the world, assembling conceptual impressions, perceiving body image, and grasping spatial relations.

Damage to one of the primary somatosensory areas of the parietal lobe will produce a loss of tactile, proprioceptive, and other sensations arising from the skin, called **hemianesthesia**. Patients are usually aware of the loss of sensation in the affected side, and do not neglect it. Damage to specific regions of the parietal lobe can also result in ignoring a part of the body or world, which is known as **hemineglect**. Patients with hemineglect can accurately perceive sensory information, but they act as if it does not exist. Their primary sensory systems such as touch, hearing, and vision, are intact, but they behave as if they only perceive information from the unaffected side. They only wash or dress one side of the body, or eat only the food on one side of the plate. Severe hemineglect may result in the patient's refusing to accept that the affected limbs even belong to them. They may even complain that someone else's leg is in bed with them.

Another condition caused by parietal lobe damage is called **astereognosis**, the inability to discriminate between objects of different shapes, textures, weights, or sizes based on touch alone. Patients with this condition, when holding an object, will be unable to identify it even though the skin receptors and nerve pathways leading up to the brain are complete and intact. Patients who cannot recognize an object by touch may still be able to draw the object and recognize the object pictured in a drawing. Similarly, **pain asymbolia** is a condition in which pain is perceived, but does not cause suffering. This usually results from injury to the brain.

■ **Learn more about the contents of this chapter** Search the Internet for *brain lobes*, *limbic system*, *homunculus*, and *Brodmann's areas*.

7 | Pain Phenomena

In normal circumstances, pain is the result of intense stimuli that are potentially or actually damaging to tissue (known as noxious stimuli). This is "good" pain that is processed and relayed by the specialized structures of the nervous system, which responds only to noxious stimuli. This **nociceptive pain** is an essential early warning device that helps protect our bodies from the environment. Nociceptive pain is caused by an injury to body tissues. Nociceptive pain is associated with such injuries as cuts, strains, sprains, bone fractures, burns, bruises, inflammation, and obstructions. Nociceptive pain is usually time-limited, so that when the tissue damage heals, pain resolves.

TYPES OF PAIN

Based on where pain is localized in the body, there are three main types of nociceptive pain—determined anatomically by which tissue type the primary nociceptive afferent has its receptive field in. These are somatic, visceral, and neuropathic pain. Any of these three types of pain can be experienced alone, or in combination with any other types. For example, some cancer patients report experiencing both somatic and visceral pain at the same time, and only a small minority of them report having neuropathic pain. All three types of pain can be experienced for shorter or longer periods of time, making them acute or chronic. Finally, different types of pain respond to different pain-reducing treatments in different ways. In general, neuropathic pain is much more difficult to treat than somatic and visceral pain.

Somatic

Somatic pain is a result of the activation of nociceptors located either in the skin (cutaneous body surface tissues) or deep tissue (musculoskeletal system). These are the most common types of pain, experienced from day to day by otherwise healthy individuals. This type of pain directly informs us, via the nervous system, of impending damage to our bodies. Typical forms of somatic skin pain include touching a hot object, injuring the skin through cutting or bruising it, scraping the skin on a rough object, or being pinched. Musculoskeletal pain is sometimes called deep somatic pain because it is more likely experienced in structures located below the surface of the skin. Structures that can give rise to musculoskeletal pain include bone, muscles, and joints. Musculoskeletal pain occurs commonly in athletes, and is another type of pain that most of us have experienced, although perhaps less frequently. It is commonly manifested as sore muscles, aching joints, or the soreness experienced during flu. Musculoskeletal pain can often be associated with quite serious medical conditions such as breaking a bone, pulling a muscle or tendon, or cramping. The quality of somatic pain can be quite different when it occurs in skin and in deep tissue, based on the types of stimuli and receptor types involved. Cutaneous pain is of the sharp and/or burning type, as opposed to the dull and throbbing, or aching type of pains of the musculoskeletal variety. Both types of somatic pain are easily localized, but musculoskeletal pain may be more diffuse, for example, along an entire muscle.

Visceral

Visceral pain is experienced in the soft internal organs of the body. These organs are enclosed within a cavity such as the thoracic (chest), abdominal, or pelvic cavity, and include the heart, lungs, stomach, intestines, liver, pancreas, kidney, bladder, and other structures. Visceral pain is caused by the activation of receptors in or on these organs, resulting from stretching, compression, or extension of the organs and/or viscera. Common causes of visceral pain can be relatively benign, such as stomachache, indigestion, or constipation, or more serious such as kidney stones, urinary tract infection, or heart attack. Unlike with somatic pain, visceral pain is not very well localized to discrete locations, and is not widely varied in its sensation. Because the density of nociceptors in the viscera is less dense than the skin, visceral pain is felt to occupy a greater area. It is typically described as dull, aching, or squeezing.

Neuropathic

Neuropathic pain is pain that is due to an inflammatory response to tissue injury, damage to a nerve or component of the nervous system, or alterations in the normal functioning of the nervous system. With neuropathic pain, the nerve fibers themselves may be dysfunctional or injured. These fibers send incorrect signals to other pain-processing centers of the nervous system. The cause of pain is abnormal, rather than being produced by somatic or visceral stimuli that are damaging the nervous system. Neuropathic pain is a syndrome in which the primary mechanism is abnormal somatosensory processing. In varieties of neuropathic pain caused by an injury, all signs of the original injury are no longer present, and the pain that the individual experiences is unrelated to the original injury or condition. With this type of pain, certain nerves continue to send pain messages to the brain even though there is no ongoing tissue damage. Examples of causes of neuropathic pain are injuries that cause nerve damage, such as squeezing or compressing the nerves of the arms or legs.

Neuropathic pain could be placed in the chronic pain category, but it has a different feel than chronic pain of a musculoskeletal nature. Neuropathic pain feels different from somatic and musculoskeletal pain and is described by individuals using the following terms: severe, sharp, lancinating, electric, stabbing, burning, cold, numbing, tingling, or causing weakness. It may have a shooting component such that it is felt to be traveling along the nerve itself up or down an arm or leg, to and from hands or feet. These sensations are quite atypical and are distinct from those experienced in somatic or visceral pain. Neuropathic pain sensations can be localized to certain regions of the body if the nerves involved are close to the skin or target organ. If the site of pain signal generation is higher up in the branching tree of nerves, a number of nerves can be affected and the pain can be felt over a wider, more diffuse area. Along these lines, in the case of a lesion in the spinal cord, pain will possibly be felt in an entire section of the body if the lesion affects the spinothalamic tract.

A number of causes of neuropathic pain exist. In some cases the underlying cause can be easily definable, while in other cases it is less obvious. Some direct causes of neuropathic pain include limb amputation, peripheral nerve injury, spinal cord injury, nerve compression, multiple sclerosis, or a tumor of a nerve. Conditions that secondarily affect the nerves that can result in neuropathic pain include alcoholism, diabetes, AIDS, or infection. Certain cancers can infiltrate the nerve, entering it and causing damage to its structure and thus its firing properties. Chemical damage of the nervous system can cause neuropathic pain, and can occur as a result of cancer treatment in the form of chemotherapy, radiation therapy, or surgery. This type of pain is severe and is described as burning or tingling, and tumors that lie close to neural structures are believed to cause the most severe pain that cancer patients experience.

Neuropathic pain is almost always associated with two sensitivity-related pain phenomena: allodynia and hyperalgesia. **Allodynia** is defined as pain resulting from a stimulus that ordinarily does not elicit a painful response. An example of such a stimulus would be touching of the skin. The underlying mechanism of allodynia is sprouting of Aβ afferent fibers into painful laminae within the spinal cord. In the noninjured state, Aβ fibers that carry impulses related to light touch, pressure, and vibration penetrate the dorsal horn and terminate in lamina III and deeper. C-fibers, small unmyelinated afferents that carry information about pain and temperature, penetrate to more superficial laminae, such as I and II. After peripheral nerve injury, there is sprouting of some Aβ afferents from lamina III into laminae I and II, while other Aβ fibers prune back their connections to synapse in laminae I–II. These afferents then are able to make connections to neurons in these laminae, which interpret the nonpainful impulses as pain signals.

Hyperalgesia is defined as an increased sensitivity to a normally painful stimulus such that it becomes painful at a lowered intensity or threshold (Figure 7.1). An example of this would be the sensation of scalding water when putting one's hand into lukewarm water. In the case of damage to the nerves of the skin, primary hyperalgesia is hyperalgesia that occurs directly at the site of injury. It is caused by the sensitization of C-fibers. Secondary hyperalgesia, the expansion of the painful zone of the skin into undamaged territory surrounding the injury site, is caused by sensitization of dorsal horn neurons that are receiving increased afferent barrage from the skin.

Hypersensitivity

The pain-processing component of the nervous system needs to be sensitive enough to detect potentially harmful stimuli. Increased sensitivity to pain after an injury helps healing by ensuring that contact with, or disruption of, injured tissue is

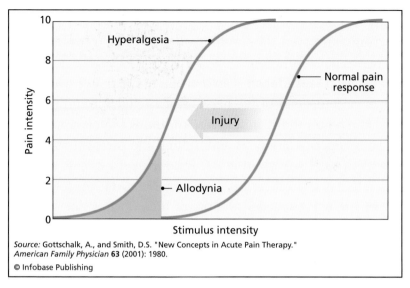

Source: Gottschalk, A., and Smith, D.S. "New Concepts in Acute Pain Therapy." *American Family Physician* **63** (2001): 1980.

© Infobase Publishing

Figure 7.1 Noxious stimuli can sensitize the nervous system response to subsequent stimuli. The normal pain response as a function of stimulus intensity is depicted by the curve at the right, where even strong stimuli are not experienced as pain. However, a traumatic injury can shift the curve to the left. Then, noxious stimuli become more painful (hyperalgesia) and typically painless stimuli are experienced as pain (allodynia).

minimized until repair is complete. In this case, increased pain sensitivity is beneficial. But in neuropathic pain states, the nervous system becomes too sensitive, causing or creating pain that does not alert the body to genuine or potential tissue damage. Pain hypersensitivity may persist for long periods after an injury has healed, or may occur in the absence of any injury. In this case, the perceived pain provides no benefit, and is a manifestation of pathological change in the nervous system.

The underlying bases of neuropathic pain include peripheral or central nerve sensitization. Following injury to a peripheral nerve by crush, stretch, or cutting, for example, sensitization occurs. A neuron begins to fire spontaneously without stimulation of its peripheral receptor, its firing threshold becomes lowered, and when activated its response to a given stimulus is greatly increased. The combination of these effects leads to increased pain sensation.

Peripheral sensitization is an increase in the responsiveness of the nociceptors end of the nerve, and a reduction in threshold of that receptor to fire in response to stimulation. It contributes to pain hypersensitivity at and around the site of tissue damage. Peripheral sensitization occurs due to the release of various inflammatory chemical mediators (i.e., ATP, prostaglandin E_2, histamine) released at the site of injury, which increase the responsiveness of nociceptors.

Damage to peripheral nerves beyond the level of the receptor can also result in a phenomenon called **ectopic discharge**, whereby nerves produce action potentials without stimulation of their receptors. Ectopic discharges can occur directly at the site of injury, in the cell bodies within the dorsal root ganglion, or in areas along axons where myelin is lost. The abnormal expression of different types of sodium channels at these sites is thought to underlie the generation of ectopic discharges. Sodium channels not found in normal nerves appear to be expressed in the injured axon, and contribute to its hyperexcitability.

Central sensitization is an increase in the spontaneous and evoked firing activity of neurons in the spinal cord dorsal horn following high levels of activity of nociceptive afferents. Although the pain feels as if it originates in the periphery, it is actually caused by neuropathic changes in sensory processing within the central nervous system itself. In this case, normal or exaggerated inputs from the periphery are able to produce abnormal levels of spinal pain signaling. Central sensitization results in biochemical and structural changes within dorsal horn nociceptive circuitry that enable it to amplify inputs and to become more excitable. These changes are typically triggered by a burst of activity in nociceptors, such as that produced after injury, which alter the strength of synaptic connections between the nociceptor and the neurons of the spinal cord.

Repetitive stimulation of C-fibers can result in prolonged discharge of spinal cord dorsal horn neurons. This phenomenon, called wind-up, is a progressive increase in the number of action potentials elicited per stimulus that occurs in dorsal horn neurons. Repetitive episodes of **wind-up** may precipitate another process called **long-term potentiation**, which involves a long-lasting increase in the strength of synaptic transmission. Wind-up is thought to last only minutes, but long-term potentiation lasts at least one hour and perhaps even days, weeks, or months. Both wind-up and long-term potentiation are thought to be part of the sensitization process involved in many chronic pain states. This strengthening of synaptic connections and firing ability is known as activity-dependent synaptic plasticity and is analogous to what happens in the brain during the formation of memories and learning.

TIME COURSE OF PAIN

The experience of pain can either be short-lived and present during direct stimulation of the nociceptor, or can last for a period longer than the actual stimulus. Some pains continue indefinitely after the injury or stimulation has subsided. **Acute pain** is temporary and short-lasting. It may last from just a few seconds to a few months as the cause of the pain heals or the stimulus is removed. Acute pain is pain that is directly related to tissue damage. It can increase in intensity over time, or it can occur intermittently, waxing and waning based on sometimes unidentifiable causes. Acute pain is easily described and observed by the individual experiencing it. Acute pain serves a protective biological function by acting as a warning of ongoing tissue damage. It is a symptom of a disease process experienced in or around the injured or diseased tissue, and is nociceptive in nature (occurring secondary to chemical, mechanical and thermal stimulation of Aδ and C-polymodal nociceptors). Causes of acute pain include touching a hot stove, scraping the skin, labor, and operations.

The longer that pain persists, the more susceptible it is to developing into a chronic pain state. As healing is completed after an injury, for example, the pain and sensitivity associated with the injury will usually resolve. But some individuals will continue to experience pain without an obvious injury, or will suffer prolonged pain that persists for months or years after the initial injury. This pain condition can be neuropathic in nature. Chronic neuropathic pain involves damage either to the peripheral or central nervous system. Rather than the nervous system functioning properly to alert the body to real or potential injury, the nervous system is malfunctioning and becomes the cause of the pain. **Chronic pain** is due to an identifiable pain generator, and is defined as pain lasting for more than three months. It is much more subjective and not as easily described as acute pain, and does not serve a biological function. Rather than being the symptom of injury or disease, chronic pain is itself a disease. Chronic pain is unrelenting and can persist for years and even decades after the initial injury. Various musculoskeletal, reproductive, gastrointestinal, and urological disorders may also cause or contribute to chronic pain.

■ **Learn more about the contents of this chapter** Search the Internet for *neuropathic pain*, *chronic pain*, and *hyperalgesia*.

8 Pain Disorders

Ongoing severe pain is recognized as a major public health problem in the United States. It is estimated that pain disorders affect 15 percent to 33 percent of the U.S. population, or as many as 100 million people. Approximately 50 million people in the United States are disabled partially or totally due to chronic pain associated with disease or illness. Chronic pain disables more people than cancer or heart disease, and costs more than both combined. It is estimated that pain costs an estimated $70 billion a year in medical costs, lost working days, and workers' compensation.

There are many diseases or medical problems that are associated with chronic pain. These include **arthritis**, **fibromyalgia**, low back pain, peripheral nerve injury, and spinal cord injury. Phantom limb pain is also considered to be a chronic pain disorder.

ARTHRITIS

More than 40 million people in the United States suffer from some form of arthritis, and many have chronic pain as a result. Arthritis is a degenerative disease that causes joint inflammation, which causes painful stiffness and swelling of the joints (Figure 8.1). There are two common forms of arthritis: osteoarthritis and rheumatoid arthritis. Osteoarthritis is a form of arthritis associated with the wearing away and degeneration

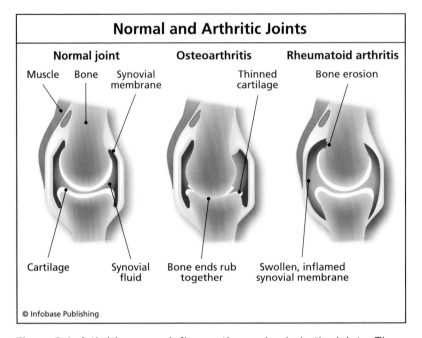

Normal and Arthritic Joints

Normal joint   **Osteoarthritis**   **Rheumatoid arthritis**

Muscle   Bone   Synovial membrane   Thinned cartilage   Bone erosion

Cartilage   Synovial fluid   Bone ends rub together   Swollen, inflamed synovial membrane

© Infobase Publishing

Figure 8.1 Arthritis causes inflammation and pain in the joints. There are two types of arthritis: osteoarthritis and rheumatoid arthritis. In the illustration above, arthritic joints are compared to a normal joint.

of the protective caps of cartilage in joints, and is associated with secondary changes in the underlying bones. This can cause pain and may impair function of the joint, most commonly in the hips, knees, and thumbs. Rheumatoid arthritis is a chronic and destructive form of joint inflammation that is caused by the body's own immune system attacking the joint tissues. A normal joint is surrounded by a protective fluid-filled joint capsule and cartilage that covers and cushions the ends of the bones. In rheumatoid arthritis, the immune system attacks the body's own tissues inside the joint capsule. White blood cells that are part of immune response enter the joint space and cause inflammation, which results in warmth, redness, swelling, and pain. During the inflammatory process, the cells of the joint also divide abnormally, resulting in a joint that is swollen and painful to the touch.

The pain of arthritis may be from any of the tissue types that are damaged in arthritis, such as the tissue that lines the joints, tendons, or ligaments. A combination of damage to any of these tissues contributes to the intensity of the pain. Swelling within the joint, the amount of heat or redness present, and damage that has occurred within the joint, all contribute to pain.

Relief of pain associated with arthritis is achieved by short- and long-term treatments. For immediate relief of rheumatoid pain, nonsteroidal anti-inflammatory drugs (**NSAIDs**) work to reduce pain caused by inflammation of the joint. These drugs do not work as well in cases of osteoarthritis because the amounts of inflammation are less. Corticosteroids, which are hormones used to reduce inflammation and pain, are also very powerful drugs and must be used carefully. Disease-modifying anti-rheumatic drugs are also used to treat rheumatoid arthritis pain. These drugs influence the immune response itself and correct abnormalities that cause the inflammatory reaction. Weight loss and low-impact exercise can also have profound effects on reducing arthritis pain.

FIBROMYALGIA

Fibromyalgia is a chronic illness that causes widespread muscle and skeletal aching, pain and stiffness, soft tissue tenderness, general fatigue, and sleep disturbances. Individuals with fibromyalgia have tender points on the body that are exquisitely sensitive to stimulation. Fibromyalgia patients experience a range of symptoms of varying intensities that come and go over time. Because its symptoms are common and generalized, and results of laboratory tests are generally normal, fibromyalgia was historically thought to be a disorder of the mind. However, recent research has proven that fibromyalgia does indeed exist. The cause is likely a dysfunction in the processing of somatosensory signals by the nervous system. Amplification of painful and non-painful sensory afferent input is likely due to abnormally low levels of serotonin and increased levels of substance P in the spinal cord, low levels of blood flow to the thalamus, and hypothalamic-pituitary-adrenal axis underfunctioning. In a large percentage of patients, the onset is triggered by an illness or injury that causes trauma to the body. Although this disorder affects about 4 million people in the United States, the vast majority are women in their mid-30s to late 50s.

The pain of fibromyalgia is profound, widespread, and chronic. It is not restricted to specific parts of the body, and can migrate to different parts of the body with varying intensity. The most common sites of pain include the neck, back, shoulders, pelvic girdle, and hands, but any body part can be involved. Pain is described by fibromyalgia sufferers as deep muscular aching, throbbing, twitching, stabbing, and shooting pain. Neurological complaints such as numbness, tingling, and burning are often present and add to the discomfort of the patient.

Treatment of fibromyalgia pain is performed with traditional NSAIDs or aspirin. In some cases, a physician may prescribe low doses of **antidepressants** that mimic the effects of serotonin, or prolong its biochemical action, or benzodiazepines, which help boost levels of serotonin in the brain and spinal cord.

LOWER BACK PAIN

Many people (70 to 85 percent) experience back pain at some time in their life, and back pain is the most frequent cause of activity limitation in people younger than 45 years old. This high percentage should not be a surprise given that the lower back supports most of the weight of the body, and the stability of the back is dependent on the sensitive anatomical components that are susceptible to damage.

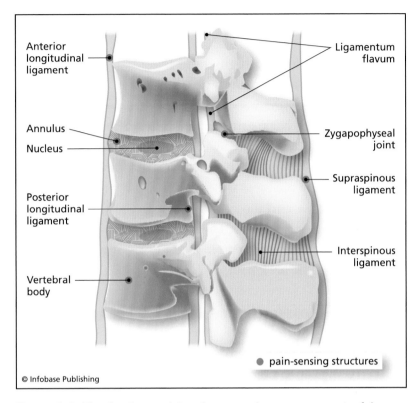

Figure 8.2 The back consists of a complex arrangement of bones, muscle, nerves, and ligaments. Pain-sensing structures help protect the back from excessive damage or stress.

There are many ways in which the back can be injured or damaged. Consider that the back is made up of 24 bones (excluding 5 fused vertebrae making up the sacrum), including those in the neck and chest areas, which are held together by a network of ligaments and muscles. In between these structures are major nerves traveling in and out of the spinal cord, vertebral disks that act as shock absorbers, and joints. The intricate arrangement of all of these structures, and their ability to move slightly with the body, make individual elements of the back susceptible to damage. Ligaments are easily sprained, muscles can be strained, discs can be ruptured, and joints can become irritated (Figure 8.2). Coupled with our active lifestyles and high-speed lives, the possibilities for injury, and pain, are enormous.

Currently, more than $50 billion is spent on the diagnosis and treatment of back pain in the United States. Pain of the lower back is treated mainly by reducing the inflammation and irritation of structures in the back. NSAIDs and anti-inflammatory drugs are the most widely accepted forms of treatment, although exercise and physical therapy are also very effective. Surgery aimed at treating pain by removing and replacing faulty disks, or making tunnels for pinched nerves, is a more serious option for chronic back pain.

PERIPHERAL NEUROPATHY

Peripheral neuropathy describes damage to the peripheral nervous system structures that transmit sensory information from the periphery to the spinal cord and brain. The population prevalence of peripheral neuropathy is about 2,400 per 100,000 (2.4 percent), rising with age to 8,000 per 100,000 individuals (8 percent).

Peripheral nerves are fragile and easily injured, and damage interferes with the communication between the skin or viscera, and the brain. Acquired peripheral neuropathies are caused by disease processes, tumors, injury from external events, alcoholism, infections, or autoimmune disorders. Examples of traumatic injuries that can produce peripheral neuropathy include cutting or crushing a nerve, or the tearing of a nerve from its location in the body. Inherited forms of peripheral neuropathy can be caused by genetic mutations.

Peripheral nerves exhibit a few distinct reactions to an insult or disease that can result in pain. After a physical injury of a nerve, degeneration results in a dying back of the nerve fibers.

At the injured end of individual axons, a structure called a **neuroma** may form. A neuroma consists of a tangled cluster of fibers that can be spontaneously active and produce ectopic discharges, which are inappropriate action potentials in the absence of stimulation. In other cases, degeneration of the insulating coat of myelin that surrounds axons can occur, leaving the nerve vulnerable to mechanical stimulation and inflammation. During demyelination, axons react by producing an abnormal population of sodium channels that further enable them to create abnormal ectopic discharges. Since the population of axons within a sensory nerve is mostly nociceptive, it is most likely that ectopic discharges will be interpreted by the spinal cord and brain as abnormal pain.

Symptoms depend on which sensory nerve is injured, but generally are experienced as pain, numbness, tingling, burning, or loss of sensation. In most cases there is a gradual onset of allodynia and hyperalgesia. The skin is extremely sensitive to objects that were once non-painful, and thresholds for what is considered painful are lowered. Pain associated with a peripheral neuropathy often comes and goes, but includes burning pain; sharp, jabbing, or electric-like pain; and extreme sensitivity to any form of stimulation.

Treatment of peripheral neuropathy begins with medications such as nonsteroidal anti-inflammatory drugs (NSAIDs), but stronger medications are necessary in most cases. Anti-seizure medications that block the action of sodium channels are very effective treatments, acting by reducing ectopic or excessive discharging. Local anesthetics that block the propagation of action potentials in the nerve, such as lidocaine, are also used, but their effects are short-lasting. Antidepressant drugs that target nociceptive circuitry within the spinal cord and brain, acting on serotonin, work well. In cases of severe pain, opioids may be prescribed.

SPINAL CORD INJURY

Damage to the spinal cord produces chronic neuropathic pain in more than 65 percent of injured individuals. Pain after spinal cord injury typically is manifested at and below the level of the injury itself. Injury of the thoracic region would thus produce pain in a girdle region around the chest, as well as in the lower extremities and feet. Pain is typically caused by mechanical injury to the spinal cord itself, or its surrounding structures, similar to that seen in lower back pain.

Compression or entrapment of nerve roots entering the spinal cord results in lancinating, burning, or stabbing pain in the skin dermatome associated with the territory of that root. The pain occurs at the level of the injury and is usually present from the time of injury onward. Injury to the spinal cord itself is perceived more diffusely in regions below the level of injury and is present on both sides of the body. It is often referred to as deafferentation pain, dysesthetic pain, or central dysesthesia syndrome. Patients commonly describe this form of pain as burning, tingling, numbness, aching, and throbbing, and report that it is usually constant in duration. It can be present in discrete regions such as a hand or finger, or an entire arm or leg. This type of pain can be both mechanical and thermal, and when thermal in nature can be felt as burning heat or freezing cold. It is not triggered by easily identifiable factors such as certain skin stimuli. Pain often occurs at the border of skin with normal sensation and skin that is insensate, and is referred to as transition zone pain. The pain occurs within a band of two to four dermatome segments, and can be localized to one or both sides of the body. Visceral pain may also be present after spinal cord injury, and is described as burning or cramping pain.

Spinal cord injury results in the interruption of descending inhibitory pain controls, such as the endogenous opioid system as well as the serotonin system. Since these systems normally suppress the communication of pain signals to the brain, their interruption enables afferent signals to travel to the brain for processing unchecked. Coupled with reconfiguration and rewiring of spinal cord sensory circuitry that permits normally non-painful signals to be translated into pain signals, spinal cord injury sets up a very strong mechanism that underlies chronic neuropathic pain.

Pain after spinal cord injury is treated in ways similar to pain from peripheral neuropathy, because it is pain of a neuropathic origin. This means that stronger compounds such as antiepileptics, channel blockers, and opiates are the preferred treatment. In some cases, pain can be relieved by surgical interruption of ascending spinal cord tracts or spinal cord stimulation.

PHANTOM LIMB PAIN

In the case of **phantom limb pain**, pain is experienced from where an amputated limb used to be. The pain is reported as squeezing of the hand or foot, burning, or crushing, and often differs from any sensation previously experienced. One patient reported that his missing hand felt like it was being crushed in a vise. In the case of an amputated leg, pain is typically experienced in the toes, ankle, and foot. After amputation of the arm, pain is felt in the fingers and hand. This is because receptor density is highest in the fingers and toes, and consequentially there are more axons per area of nerve that are dedicated to carrying these signals.

Phantom limb pain cannot be caused by something stimulating the missing body part; rather, it must be caused by an alteration in the functioning in the nervous system above the site where the limb was amputated. In this case, inappropriate nerve signals are generated at the site where the peripheral nerve was cut. Due to the labeled line system where individual nerve fibers course through the spinal cord and thalamus to specific targets in the brain, inappropriate firing from an interrupted fiber still reaches the brain in its original area, despite not originating in the skin. The brain does not realize this and assigns the pain signal to the missing part of the body. There is also evidence for altered nervous activity within the brain as a result of the loss of sensory input from the amputated limb.

Phantom limb pain is generally intractable and chronic. Once it develops, such pain persists and is rarely improved by conventional medical treatments, and destructive surgical procedures are also of limited use. One effective treatment, developed recently by neuroscientist V.S. Ramachandran, uses a mirror box to trick the brain of phantom limb patients. Patients with amputations of the arm and phantom limb pain place their arms inside a box with an angled mirror that reverses the image of an intact arm to the amputated side. To the patient looking down at the boxes, it appears as if they have two arms. Moving the remaining arm in the box fools the brain into thinking that the amputated arm is present and moving. This reduces the patient's phantom pain. It is hypothesized that artificially linking the visual and motor system in the parietal lobe helps patients to create a coherent body image, and reduce pain as a result of incompatible input.

■ **Learn more about the contents of this chapter**   Search the Internet for *rheumatoid arthritis, corticosteroids,* and *V.S. Ramachandran.*

9 | Endogenous Pain Control

The nervous system is remarkable in the way it deals with incoming nociceptive signals. It is thought that there is a direct relationship between pain signals and experienced pain intensity, but in some cases, this relationship can be highly variable. This variability depends on the status of the nervous system and how it processes incoming sensory signals. For example, touch, which is not normally a painful stimulus, can be changed such that its threshold to induce pain is lowered dramatically. Touching an area of skin after inflammation or tissue damage is extremely painful. Similarly, changes in mental state can cause changes in perceived pain intensity. Factors such as arousal, emotional stress, attention, and relaxation, all of which involve central nervous system mechanisms, can greatly influence pain perception. The most extreme of these is exemplified by traumatic injuries sustained during combat or sporting events. Initially, very severe and life-threatening injuries are reported as relatively painless by the individual, whereas in other circumstances the injuries would be extremely painful. Here, pain responses are modified due to mechanisms that activate the nervous system's internal pain control network.

This so-called endogenous pain control system is the way in which pain signals can be modulated at different levels of the nervous system by anatomical and biochemical means. Several mechanisms of pain control are now identified. These include the descending inhibitory control network and endogenous opioid systems.

DESCENDING REGULATION OF PAIN

The brain is capable of modifying nociceptive signals before they reach it. Experiments in the early 1950s demonstrated that supraspinal sites (those above the spinal cord) play a role in controlling ascending pain information traveling up from the spinal cord. It was shown that in cats in which the connections between the brain and spinal cord had been interrupted, cells in the spinal cord dorsal horn became more responsive to painful stimulation of the hindpaw. These results provided the first clues that supraspinal control of pain was inhibitory in nature, and that this inhibition was continuously active.

The idea that descending brain stem systems can modify pain signals in the spinal cord is supported by evidence gained from a therapeutic technique called stimulation-produced analgesia. **Stimulation-produced analgesia** is a method whereby small brain sites are stimulated electrically through fine electrodes, resulting in suppression of nociceptive signaling. In humans and other animals, stimulation-produced analgesia does not affect non-painful sensation, movement, or awareness. Two important observations were obtained from this technique: (1) nociceptive neurons in the spinal cord could be selectively inhibited by stimulating a brain stem site called the periaqueductal gray; and (2) lesions interrupting a region of the spinal cord called the dorsolateral funiculus, which contains a number of white matter fiber tracts, could inhibit the effects of stimulation-produced analgesia.

The effective location of stimulation-produced analgesia is the **periaqueductal gray**. Found in the midbrain, it is a sleeve of gray matter located around the cerebral aqueduct. The periaqueductal gray receives a number of strong inputs from the hypothalamus, a region of the brain involved in maintaining body homeostasis, the frontal and insular cortex, and the amygdala. These latter brain regions are involved in processing awareness and emotion. The major source of input to the periaqueductal gray is from the spinal cord, particularly from lamina I nociceptive neurons.

Fibers of the periaqueductal gray project downward to a set of nuclei called the raphe nuclei that reside in an adjacent region of the brain stem called the rostral ventromedial medulla. The raphe nuclei are a collection of a number of small nuclei, the largest of which is the raphe magnus. The raphe nuclei produce the neurotransmitter serotonin, and are considered to contain the major output neurons of the descending pain inhibition system. Projections from this region are sent forward and upward toward the cortex, as well as down into the spinal cord.

Raphaespinal fibers course downward in the spinal cord in the dorsolateral funiculus, a region of white matter axon pathways just outside of the dorsal horn of the gray matter, and make connections directly onto neurons in the superficial spinal dorsal horn. Connections are made along the entire length of the spinal cord, but are especially dense in regions receiving high densities of sensory afferent fibers, such as the cervical and lumbar enlargements that receive inputs from the arms and legs. Fibers synapse directly onto second-order nociceptive neurons that make up the spinothalamic pain pathway, as well as local inhibitory interneurons that modulate the excitability of a number of types of pain-processing

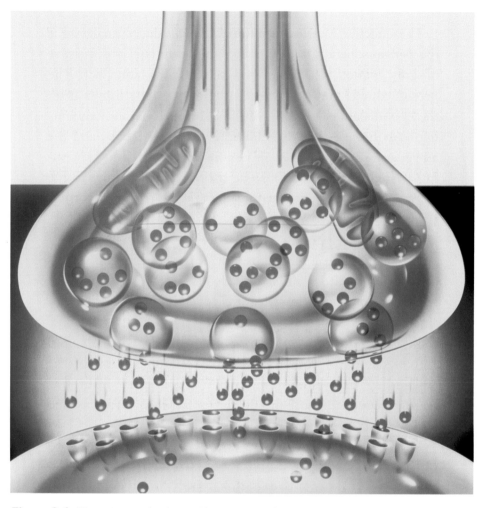

Figure 9.1 Neurotransmitters, such as serotonin, are released from vesicles (blue spheres) when an electrical signal reaches the end of an axon. The neurotransmitters (red) travel across a junction, known as a synapse, and attach to receptors on the membrane of an adjacent nerve cell.

neurons within the dorsal horn. Inhibitory interneurons are interspersed among dorsal horn pain-receiving and pain-processing neurons, and can strongly modulate the excitability of neurons in the substantia gelatinosa region of the spinal cord that receives the majority of pain projections from the periphery.

Raphaespinal fibers utilize serotonin as a neurotransmitter to dampen the activity of these neurons. Serotonin is released by descending fibers and binds to specific serotonin receptors on nociceptive neurons (Figure 9.1). Binding causes a generalized inhibitory effect on pain transmission through receptors that block the firing of nociceptive neurons directly, or by binding to receptors that excite interneurons, which in turn indirectly inhibit the firing of nociceptive neurons. Serotoninergic innervation of the spinal cord is provided only by raphaespinal fibers.

OPIOID ANALGESIA

Extremely potent pain-killing drugs, such as morphine or heroin, administered into specific regions of the brain, produce a strong pain-reducing response. These drugs do not take effect through peripheral receptors in the skin, but on receptors in the central nervous system. Anatomical sites in the brain where administration is effective in reducing pain are the same as those activated in stimulation-produced analgesia, the periaqueductal gray and rostroventral medulla. Direct injection of these drugs into the cerebral ventricle that the periaqueductal gray surrounds produces a short-lasting analgesia. Analgesia during injury or other stressful situations results in the release of one or more opioid peptides in the midbrain and other regions. Stimuli that can cause opiate release in the periaqueductal gray include pain stimuli ascending from the spinal cord and from higher centers of the brain.

The brain produces its own natural morphine-like small peptide molecules called **endogenous opioids**. The three most potent classes of endogenous opioids are the endorphins, enkephalins, and dynorphins. These molecules bind to opioid receptors in the brain and spinal cord. The word endorphin itself is abbreviated from "endogenous morphine." The best-known endorphins are α-, β-, and ϒ-endorphin, of which β-endorphin appears to be most implicated in pain relief. Each of these molecules is derived from one of three genes that encode a large precursor molecule that is cut up by enzymes into active opioid molecule peptide fragments. These are propiomelanocortin for β-endorphin, proenkephalin for enkephalin, and prodynorphin for dynorphin.

Opioids act by stimulating the opioid receptors termed mu, delta, and kappa. Specific classes of receptors have been described for each type of opiate. These are called μ (mu) for morphine-sensitive receptors, ε (epsilon) for β-endorphin, δ (delta) for enkephalins, and κ (kappa) for dynorphin. These receptors have subtly different roles in pain inhibition. Although the anatomical distribution of the opioid peptides differs, members of each family are located at sites associated with the processing of pain signals in the nervous system, and the distribution of the large endogenous opioid precursor molecules generally parallels the location of the opioid receptors. Neurons containing enkephalin and dynorphin are found in the periaqueductal gray and rostroventral medulla, as well as in the spinal cord dorsal horn. Their density within the spinal cord is particularly high in the superficial laminae I and II. β-endorphin has a more limited distribution, however, and is found mainly in neurons of the hypothalamus that project to the periaqueductal gray. High levels of the mu receptor are found in the periaqueductal gray region and in the superficial dorsal horn of the spinal cord, like the enkephalin-containing neurons.

Drugs that bind to the various opioid receptors produce different effects in response to different types of pain. Drugs

An Example of Stress-induced Analgesia

There are many descriptions of stress-induced analgesia, where during a particularly traumatic injury or event, individuals become insensitive to pain in a situation that should be extremely painful. One such report comes from the writings of David Livingstone, a Scottish explorer traveling through Africa.

> I heard a shout. Starting, and looking half round, I saw the lion just in the act of springing upon me. I was upon a little height; he caught my shoulder as he sprang, and we both came to the ground below together. Growling horribly close to my ear, he shook me as a terrier dog does a rat. The shock produced a stupor similar to that which seems to be felt by a mouse after the first shake of the cat. It caused a sort of dreaminess, in which there was no sense of pain nor feeling of terror, though [I was] quite conscious of all that was happening. It was like what patients partially under the influence of chloroform describe, who see all the operation, but feel not the knife. The shake annihilated fear, and allowed no sense of horror in looking round at the beast. This peculiar state is probably produced in all animals killed by the carnivora; and if so, is a merciful provision by our benevolent Creator for lessening the pain of death.

Livingstone, David. Missionary Travels and Researches in South Africa, 1857 that bind to kappa receptors inhibit nociceptive responses after painful mechanical stimulation of the skin, whereas compounds that act on mu receptors are the most effective in reducing responses to painful thermal stimuli. Different classes of opiate receptors may therefore modulate specific types of painful information.

The opioids activate descending inhibitory pathways beginning in the periaqueductal gray. The activation of these pathways is thought to suppress the activity of spinal cord interneurons that release the inhibitory neurotransmitter GABA. GABA normally inhibits the activity of descending inhibitory control pathways. So in this configuration, opiates release these pathways from GABAergic inhibition, increasing activity in the descending pathways and thus suppressing pain, a process called **disinhibition**. GABA exerts its effect by binding to specific receptors that essentially increase the polarization of neuronal membranes. This hyperpolarization makes it more difficult for a neuron to fire.

Opioids also exert a direct effect on spinal cord nociceptive neurons. The predominant spinal opioid receptors present in lamina I are mu and delta, and in laminae II to V, kappa. Just as with the periaqueductal gray, injection of opiates into the space surrounding the spinal cord results in reduction in nociceptive transmission. Interneurons in the superficial dorsal horn that contain high levels of enkephalin and dynorphin lie in close proximity to the terminals of nociceptive afferents and the dendrites of second-order dorsal horn neurons that receive afferent input. Mu receptors are located both on the presynaptic fiber terminals and post-synaptic projection neurons, and act by inhibiting the release of glutamate and substance P from primary nociceptors' afferent sites. Postsynaptically, opiates act to suppress the firing activity of nociceptive neurons by hyperpolarizing their neuronal membranes. This multi-site action of opioids demonstrates their high importance in the inhibition of pain signal transmission.

■ **Learn more about the contents of this chapter** Search the Internet for *opioid receptors*, *analgesia*, and *pain control*.

10 Exogenous Pain Treatments

The management of pain is a high priority among those who suffer and health care providers alike. For thousands of years, doctors have been relieving the pain of their patients with a wide variety of medications and treatments. Ancient civilizations left records on stone tablets about how pain was to be treated: pressure, heat, water, and sun. Early humans related pain to evil, magic, and possession by demons, and the treatment of pain was left to shamans who used herbs, rites, and ceremonies as treatments.

Modern interventions for reducing pain target any structure or chemical event along the pathway that participates in the transmission of pain signals from the receptor level to the final endpoint, the brain. The complex nature of the pain system affords many opportunities for the modulation or interruption of pain signal transmission by a number of approaches. At the level of the peripheral nociceptor, local anesthetics and anti-inflammatory drugs target the nociceptor activation and the generation of pain impulses in nociceptive nerves. The peripheral nerve is another target, with local anesthetic drugs that specifically block nociceptive impulses along axons. Dorsal root ganglion cell bodies are targeted by local anesthetics as well. Once in the spinal cord, nociceptive impulses can be modulated by local anesthetics that block neuronal transmission of signals, and opioids and

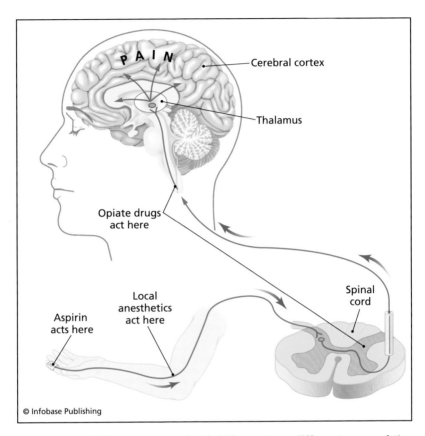

Figure 10.1 Different types of painkillers act on different areas of the nervous system. Aspirin acts by reducing pain signals in the distant peripheral nerves, such as those in the finger. Local anesthetics block pain signals traveling up the nerve, while opioids manage pain processing in the brain and spinal cord.

other compounds can be used to activate inhibitory neurons that dampen pain signals or inhibit nociceptive neurons directly. Opioids and related compounds also are effective in managing pain processing within the brain (Figure 10.1).

Treatment approaches fall into several distinct classes depending on the therapeutic methodology: pharmacology, surgical lesions, stimulation, and psychotherapy. Pharmacological methodologies aim to interrupt pain signaling at a neurochemical, and often peripheral, level by using nonsteroidal anti-inflammatory drugs or opioids. Surgical lesions aim to interrupt the anatomical pathways that pain signals utilize by either physically interrupting them, or by making highly targeted lesions in pain-processing structures. Stimulation techniques attempt to activate pain-inhibiting mechanisms in the brain and spinal cord by either electrical or magnetic means. Finally, psychotherapy attempts to enable the individual sufferer to use the power of the mind to reduce the intensity and severity of the experience of pain.

DRUGS TO TREAT PAIN

The pharmacological treatment of pain utilizes pain-relieving drugs called **analgesics**.

The word analgesic is derived from ancient Greek and means to "stop pain." Analgesic refers to the class of drugs that includes most painkillers, such as nonsteroidal anti-inflammatory drugs (NSAIDs), acetaminophen, narcotics, antidepressants, and anticonvulsants. Nonprescription or over-the-counter pain relievers are generally used for mild to moderate pain. Prescription pain relievers, sold through a pharmacy under the direction of a physician, are used for moderate to severe pain.

Non-narcotic agents such as NSAIDs and acetaminophen are available as over-the-counter and prescription medications, and used to treat pain initially. Common NSAIDs include aspirin, ibuprofen, and naproxen sodium. These drugs are used to treat pain from inflammation and work by blocking production of pain-enhancing neurotransmitters and inflammatory mediators at the level of the peripheral receptor. Acetaminophen is also effective against pain, but its ability to reduce inflammation is limited. Unlike narcotics, NSAIDs do not cause the development of tolerance or physical dependence with sustained use.

NSAIDs exert their effects against inflammation by their ability to inhibit prostaglandin biosynthesis. **Prostaglandins** are fatty acid derivatives that can produce a variety of biological effects in response to trauma, including the inflammatory response. The NSAIDs do this by inhibiting an enzyme called cyclooxygenase (**COX**) that is crucial in the initial synthesis of prostaglandins. There are two major forms of the COX enzyme, COX-1 and COX-2. COX-1 regulates prostaglandins that are important for the health of the stomach lining and kidneys through mucus production, and blockade of this enzyme with an NSAID can cause stomach problems. COX-2 is an enzyme that regulates the production of prostaglandins that cause inflammation, pain, and fever. It mediates the pain of inflammation by sensitizing peripheral nociceptors. The beneficial effects of NSAIDs result from their ability to block COX-2. Most NSAIDs inhibit COX-1 more than COX-2, and as such, pharmaceutical companies have invested fortunes to produce selective COX-2 inhibitors.

Stronger pain requires the use of narcotic agents. **Narcotics** are able to lessen very intense pain effectively, and are used for acute pain that does not respond to NSAIDs and acetaminophen. Narcotic analgesics are the preferred drugs used in the treatment of severe cancer, post-surgical, labor, burn, and chronic types of pain (Figure 10.2). Opioids raise the threshold for the perception of pain, and alter an individual's reaction to pain. Thus they affect both the sensory-discriminative and motivational-affective components of pain. Patients often report that with morphine treatment, pain is still present, but they are less bothered by it. Narcotics are classified as either opiates or opioids. Opiates include the commonly used morphine and codeine. These drugs are derived from opium, a compound found in poppy plants. Opioids are a class of synthetic drugs based on the structure of opium, and include oxycodon, methadone, and meperidine. Opioids have a narcotic effect, that is, they induce sedation as well as pain relief, and some patients may become physically dependent (addicted) after long-term use. With long-term use the body develops a tolerance to narcotics, reducing

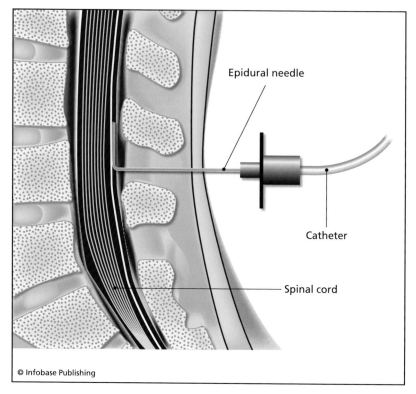

Figure 10.2 An epidural block is an injection of an anesthetic drug given into the epidural space. Epidural blocks are used to reduce pain during childbirth and various surgical procedures.

their effectiveness over time and requiring higher and higher concentrations for effectiveness.

Narcotics work by depressing nociceptive transmission at central synapses. This is achieved at the level of the spinal cord by inhibiting the release of nociceptive neurotransmitters from primary afferent terminals as well as by depressing post-synaptic activity. Thus, opiates and opioids mimic the effect of endogenous opioids released in the spinal cord upon activation by the descending inhibitory systems. In addition, activation of opioid receptors at brain stem sites, such as the periaqueductal gray, leads to the activation of descending inhibitory systems.

Antidepressants and anticonvulsants are also effective drugs for treating pain. Although originally developed to treat depression, antidepressants are also effective in combating chronic headaches, cancer pain, and pain associated with nerve damage. Antidepressants that have been shown to have analgesic properties include amitriptyline, trazodone, and imipramine. In addition, anti-anxiety drugs called benzodiazepines also act as muscle relaxants and are sometimes used as pain relievers. Originally developed to treat seizure disorders and epilepsy, **anticonvulsants** can be used to relieve pain as well. This is due to the similarities between pathophysiological mechanisms underlying both epilepsy and neuropathic pain. Sodium channel blockers act to reversibly block the generation and conduction of action potentials along nerve fibers. Their main action is to physically block the pores of sodium channels, inhibiting the flow of sodium ions through the channel that depolarizes the neuron. The degree of blockage is inversely proportional to the extent of myelination on the nerve fibers, such that nociceptive C-fibers and Aδ-fibers are blocked preferentially in comparison with thickly myelinated, non-nociceptive primary afferents. Drugs such as phenytoin and carbamazepine are effective in reducing pain associated with nerve damage.

SURGERY

In cases where analgesic drugs are ineffective in treating or managing severe pain, surgical procedures can be performed to help relieve pain. Surgery is often the best option for mechanical causes of pain such as back problems or musculoskeletal injuries, but can also be useful for anatomically interrupting pain pathways. Surgery may take the form of intentional destruction of spinal root, spinal cord, or brain tissue. In cases where spinal nerve roots are compressed resulting in pain, surgical relief involves the removal of a portion of the spinal vertebra that is causing the compression. More radical operations involving the spinal cord and its afferent roots include rhizotomy and cordotomy.

Posterior rhizotomy is the cutting of the afferent portion of a sensory nerve just before it enters the spinal cord. If pain is caused by traumatic lesions of a peripheral nerve, visceral injury, cancer, or a skin lesion in a certain area of the body, the sensory nerve that carries signals into the spinal cord is cut, and the corresponding dorsal root ganglion removed. This often brings permanent relief from pain, as well as the inability to receive other sensory information from the corresponding dermatome.

Cordotomy is a surgical procedure that interrupts nociceptive pathways in the spinal cord. When nerve fibers within the spinal cord are cut, nociceptive signals are interrupted before they reach second-order nociceptive neurons of the spinal cord or brain. Cordotomy can be performed at either the site of entry of nociceptive afferents, or above the level of entry along the pain pathway. Dorsal root entry zone cordotomy is a procedure in which a destructive lesion is created in the spinal cord just adjacent to the point of entry of afferent nerve fibers from the dorsal roots. These types of lesions are designed to destroy the initial entry point of nociceptive afferent fibers as well as superficial dorsal horn laminae (I–II) that process nociceptive signals and relay them to the brain. Anterolateral cordotomy is aimed at interrupting the communication of nociceptive impulses by the spinothalamic tract, the main pathway by which the spinal cord communicates pain information to the brain. The spinothalamic tract is located in the anterolateral quadrant of the spinal cord. Cordotomy must be done at spinal levels higher than where nociceptive signals are entering the spinal cord. Anterolateral cordotomy provides selective elimination of pain and temperature perception several segments below the spinal segment at which the lesion is placed. It is effective for unilateral, mainly somatic pain. For visceral pain or bilateral pain, two-sided cordotomies may be required. Similar to the anterolateral cordotomy is the commissural myelotomy (cutting of spinal cord tracts), whereby the fibers of the spinothalamic tract are interrupted as they cross the spinal cord in lamina X before their ascent to the brain. This procedure produces pain relief on both sides of the body, but is not widely used.

Thalamic nuclei lesions can disrupt the processing of nociceptive impulses as well, but these surgeries are rare considering the danger of opening the brain to infection, unintentionally destroying healthy brain tissue, and the success of cordotomy. In cases where it is performed, the ventral posterior lateral and ventral posterior medial nuclei are targeted for destruction. Finally, a lesion in the cingulate gyrus has been used to treat pain and severe psychiatric disorders, but is no longer performed routinely.

STIMULATION

Electrical stimulation, including **transcutaneous electrical stimulation** (**TENS**), implanted electric nerve stimulation, and deep brain or spinal cord stimulation, is quite effective in managing pain. Pain relief can be achieved by selective stimulation of particular subtypes of primary afferent nerve fibers. Afferent fibers can be activated by implanted electrodes or by natural stimuli such as vibration.

TENS uses small electrical impulses delivered by electrodes placed on the surface of the skin to stimulate Aβ fibers in nerves, resulting in pain relief during stimulation. **Peripheral nerve stimulation** uses electrodes placed surgically around peripheral nerves that can be activated by the patient to stimulate the nerve and reduce pain. This approach is beneficial when an individual peripheral nerve can be associated with localized pain. Similarly,

spinal cord stimulation involves implanting an electrode into the epidural space surrounding the spinal cord, which when activated, stimulates the spinal cord and produces pain relief. The dorsal column system is targeted, and collaterals of large Aβ fibers are activated as they ascend toward the brain. **Deep brain stimulation** is considered to be an experimental procedure, and remains viable only for managing extreme pain. Typically, electrodes are implanted into the brain that end in either the ventral posterior medial or lateral nuclei of the thalamus, or internal capsule. When activated, they stimulate pain-processing areas. The periaqueductal gray region of the midbrain is a recent target of deep brain stimulation, and renders parts of the periphery completely insensitive to pain.

PSYCHOTHERAPY

The power of the mind can also be harnessed to reduce the severity of the experience of pain. We are all familiar with the

Acupuncture for Pain Relief

Acupuncture is a traditional Chinese practice more than 2,000 years old that can provide pain relief. Acupuncture treatment consists of the insertion of thin needles into the skin at precise locations on the body, followed by gentle twirling of the needles. Acupuncture charts mapping the insertion sites of needles are highly complex, traditionally showing 361 points that lie on 14 meridians corresponding to internal organs. A variation on traditional acupuncture is electroacupuncture, in which wires are attached to the needles and electrical currents are passed through them.

phenomenon of the sensation of pain becoming more or less intense based on our state of mind. When we are distressed, anxious, or fearful, the intensity of pain can be exaggerated. For example, during a minor medical procedure that produces some small amount pain, this pain can be magnified if the patient is overly anxious. On the other hand, if the mind is calm, then the intensity of painful experiences can be lessened.

Distraction, or **cognitive refocusing**, aims to direct a person's attention and concentration at other stimuli, thereby lessening the focus on pain. These stimuli may be internal, such as thoughts, or external, such as TV. The most effective stimuli are those that are unique and changing, and those that require input from most or all of the senses at the same time—seeing, hearing, tasting, touching, and smelling. Relaxation may be used for all types of pain, but it is most effective for chronic pain. Relaxation creates a state of relative freedom from anxiety and muscle tension that can amplify pain. Relaxation methods focus on simple ideas or movements such as slow deep breathing and alternately tightening and relaxing muscles of the body.

Psychotherapy utilizing a **cognitive-behavioral approach** in the treatment of chronic pain aims to influence the way an individual thinks about pain. It recognizes the roles that cognitive factors, such as appraisal, belief, and expectation, play in exacerbating pain and suffering, contributing to disability, and influencing response to treatment. Cognitive-behavioral interventions are designed to help patients develop coping techniques and become aware of the impact that negative pain-related thoughts and feelings have on experiencing pain. The principles of cognitive-behavioral therapy are: (1) individuals are active processors of information, not passive reactors; (2) thoughts can elicit and influence mood and affect physiological processes, and the environment can alter mood and thought processes; (3) behavior is determined by both the individual and environmental factors; (4) individuals can learn more adaptive ways of thinking, feeling, and behaving; and (5) individuals can be agents in changing their maladaptive thoughts, feelings, and behaviors. Using these thought-changing techniques can help to lessen the impact of the experience of pain.

■ **Learn more about the contents of this chapter** Search the Internet for *cordotomy*, *NSAID*, and *periaqueductal gray*.

Glossary

Action potential Electrical discharge (impulse) of a neuron.

Acute pain Pain experienced in the short term.

Afferent Nerve fiber carrying information toward the central nervous system.

Allodynia Pain caused by a stimulus that does not normally cause pain.

Amygdala Brain structure involved in emotional processing.

Analgesic Pain-reducing drug.

Anticonvulsant Drug used to reduce seizures that is sometimes used to treat pain.

Antidepressants A drug used to treat depression.

Arthritis Painful inflammation of the joints.

Astereognosis Inability to discriminate between objects of different shapes, textures, weights, or sizes based on touch alone.

ATP Adenosine triphosphate, a neurotransmitter molecule.

Aα fiber Large-diameter nerve fiber that carries information regarding touch, and muscle and body position.

Aβ fiber Medium-diameter nerve fiber that carries information regarding touch.

Aδ fiber Small-diameter nerve fiber that carries information regarding pain and temperature.

Aδ mechanical nociceptor Receptor structure that receives information regarding pain.

Blood-brain barrier Protective barrier around the brain and spinal cord.

Brain Organ responsible for control of body activities and interpretation of information received from the senses.

Brodmann's areas Numbered anatomical regions of the cerebral cortex.

Calcitonin gene–related peptide (CGRP) A large peptide that is a pain neurotransmitter.

Cauda equina Nerves at the end of the spinal cord that resemble the tail of a horse.

Central sensitization Process in which sensory neurons of the spinal cord are hypersensitized.

Cerebrospinal fluid Fluid that provides nutrients and support to the brain and spinal cord.

Cervical enlargement Region of the spinal cord that innervates the arms.

C-fiber Very small–diameter nerve fiber that carries information regarding pain and temperature.

Chemoreceptors Specialized receptors that are activated by certain chemicals.

Chronic pain Long-lasting pain.

Cognitive refocusing Psychological technique used to refocus the mind onto other thoughts.

Cognitive-behavioral approach Psychological technique used to think about pain differently.

Congenital insensitivity to pain Genetic disorder in which the individual is not sensitive to painful stimuli.

Conus medullaris End point of the spinal cord.

Cordotomy Cutting of the spinal cord to reduce pain transmission.

Cortex Outermost surface of the brain, where higher-order processing occurs.

COX Enzyme responsible for contributing to inflammatory pain.

C-polymodal nociceptor Pain receptor that responds to mechanical, thermal, and chemical stimuli.

Deep brain stimulation Pain-reducing technique whereby brain structures are electrically stimulated.

Dermatome Region of the skin innervated by a single nerve.

Disinhibition The act of enhancing the firing ability of a neuron through reducing inhibitory controls.

Distension Expansion or stretching.

Dorsal column system Fiber pathway in the spinal cord that carries information regarding touch and visceral pain.

Dorsal Related to or situated near the back of an animal.

Dorsal horn Anatomical region of the spinal cord that receives sensory signals for processing and relay.

Dorsal root ganglion (DRG) Location of cell bodies from peripheral nerve fibers.

Dura mater Tough protective covering of the brain and spinal cord.

Ectopic discharge Abnormal nerve firing.

Efferent Nerve fiber carrying information away from the central nervous system.

Endogenous opioids Naturally occurring opioid peptides within the body.

Epidural space Space around the spinal cord.

Fasciculus cuneatus Spinal cord pathway carrying information from the upper body.

Fasciculus gracilis Spinal cord pathway carrying information from the lower body.

Fibromyalgia Generalized chronic pain condition.

Filum terminale Terminating fiber of the spinal cord.

GABA An inhibitory neurotransmitter.

Generator potential Signal sent from the receptor to the nerve, indicating receipt of stimulus.

Glabrous Skin of the palms of the hands and soles of the feet.

Glutamate A widespread excitatory neurotransmitter.

Glycine An inhibitory neurotransmitter.

Gray matter Region of the spinal cord and brain where cell bodies of neurons reside.

Hemianesthesia Inability to feel one side of the body.

Hemineglect Ignorance of one side of the body.

Hippocampus Brain structure involved in memory formation.

Homunculus Topographical representation of the body on the surface of the brain.

Hyperalgesia Decreased threshold to a normally painful stimulus.

Innervate To supply nerves to a body part or organ.

Intensity Action potential firing that encodes the strength of a stimulus.

Internal capsule   Fiber bundle within the brain that carries ascending and descending information from and to the body.

Interneuron   Small relay neuron involved in information processing.

Intrathecal space   Space surrounding the spinal cord filled with cerebrospinal fluid.

Labeled line   Theory explaining direct pathways from receptor to brain.

Laminae   Layers of the spinal cord gray matter.

Limbic system   Areas within the brain that are associated with the emotions.

Long-term potentiation   The ability of the nervous system to retain information and become easily activated.

Lumbar enlargement   Portion of the spinal cord that innervates the legs.

Mechanoreceptors   Receptors that respond to mechanical stimuli.

Meissner's corpuscles   Receptors that respond to fine touch and vibration.

Meninges   Membranes that cover the brain and spinal cord.

Merkel's disks   Receptors that respond to texture and rough edges.

Modality   The type of stimuli.

Monoamine   Neurotransmitter class derived from amino acids.

Motor nerves   Nerves that communicate motor signals to muscles.

Myelin   Fatty sheath that surrounds axons and enhances the speed of conduction of action potentials.

Narcotic   Strong painkilling drug based on opioids.

Neuroma   Formation on the end of a cut or damaged nerve.

Neuropathic pain   Pain with its origin in the nervous system.

Neuropeptide   Large neurotransmitter molecule that is often long-lasting.

Neurotransmitter   Molecule that signals between neurons.

NMDA   Class of receptor molecules that binds to glutamate.

Nociceptive pain   Pain in response to a damaging or potentially damaging stimulus.

Nociceptors   Receptors that respond to pain and noxious temperatures.

Node of Ranvier   Break in the myelin sheath surrounding axons.

Norepinephrine   Excitatory neurotransmitter involved in pain processing.

Noxious   Harmful or destructive.

NSAID   Nonsteroidal anti-inflammatory drug used to combat inflammatory pain.

Nucleus cuneatus   Nucleus in the brain stem that receives sensory information from the upper body.

Nucleus gracilis   Nucleus in the brain stem that receives sensory information from the lower body.

Oligodendrocytes   Myelin-producing cells of the central nervous system.

Opioids   Natural and artificial class of highly potent painkillers.

Opponent code   Variable signaling pattern of action potentials.

Pacinian corpuscles   Receptors that respond to touch, vibration, or other sensory stimuli.

Pain asymbolia   Condition, caused by damage to the brain, in which pain is perceived but does not cause suffering.

Pain threshold   The level at which a stimulus becomes painful to the body.

Pain tolerance   The amount of pain an individual can withstand.

Parietal association area   Area of the brain that assimilates a large number of sensory inputs.

Parietal lobe   Area of the brain involved in interpreting the world.

Periaqueductal gray   Brain stem region that is the source of descending inhibitory pain controls.

Peripheral nerve   Nerve outside of the spinal cord.

Peripheral nerve stimulation   Electrical stimulation of the peripheral nerves in an attempt to reduce pain.

Peripheral sensitization   Overresponsiveness of peripheral nerves to stimulation.

Phantom limb pain   Pain in an amputated limb caused by changes in the brain and spinal cord.

Plexus   Network of nerve fibers.

Polysynaptic   Pertaining to a chain of neurons.

Posterior rhizotomy   Cutting of the afferent portion of a sensory nerve just before it enters the spinal cord.

Primary afferent fibers   Incoming sensory fibers entering the spinal cord.

Primary afferent neuron   Peripheral afferent nerve that transmits information from peripheral receptors to the spinal cord.

Primary sensory cortex   Brain region that receives incoming sensory information from the thalamus.

Proprioception   The sensation of the location of the body and limbs in space.

Prostaglandin   An enzyme involved in the inflammatory pain response.

Raphe nuclei   Brain stem nuclei that produce the neurotransmitter serotonin.

Raphaespinal tract   Pathway that extends from the raphe nuclei to the spinal cord and carries serotonin.

Receptive field   Area of the skin where the ending of a nerve fiber is sensitive.

Referred pain   Pain experienced on the skin near injured viscera.

Reflex arc   Simple pathway involving a few neurons that control a reflex.

Ruffini endings   Receptors that respond to stretching of the skin.

Saltatory conduction   Jumping conduction of action potentials from node to node along an axon.

Schwann cells   Myelin-producing cells of the peripheral nervous system.

Secondary sensory cortex   Region of the brain that performs more complex processing of sensory signals.

Sensory nerves   Nerves that convey information regarding sensory stimuli.

Sensory receptor   Receptor that receives sensory information.

Sensory transduction   The conversion of thermal or other stimuli into electrical impulses.

Serotonin   An inhibitory neurotransmitter involved in pain processing.

Signal encoding Process whereby information is encoded in the pattern of action potential impulses.

Somatic pain Pain of the skin and muscles.

Somatotopic Organizational pattern related to the accurate arrangement of the body.

Spatial code Coding of information regarding location of stimuli.

Spinal cord Extension of the brain that carries sensory and motor commands to and from the body.

Spinal cord stimulation Electrical stimulation of the spinal cord that aims to reduce pain.

Spinal nerves Nerves exiting and entering the spinal cord.

Spinothalamic tract Major tract of the spinal cord that carries information related to pain and temperature to the thalamus.

Stimulation-produced analgesia Stimulation of brain regions aimed at reducing pain.

Substance P Neurotransmitter involved in pain processing.

Tactile resolution The ability to detect fine differences in the size of an object.

Temporal code Coding of the length of stimulation.

Thalamus Major relay center between the spinal cord and brain.

Tracts Pathways in the central nervous system composed of axons in the white matter.

Transcutaneous electrical stimulation (TENS) Skin stimulation aimed at reducing pain transmission.

Ventral Related to or situated near the front or belly of an animal.

Ventral horn Anatomical region of the spinal cord that sends output signals to muscles for movement.

Vertebrae Bones that surround and protect the spinal cord and roots.

Viscera Internal organs and their membranes.

Visceral pain Pain originating in the internal organs of the body.

White matter Region of the spinal cord made up of axons traveling up and down.

Wind-up Consecutive stimuli causing increased sensitivity of spinal cord neurons.

Bibliography

Abdulla, F.A., T.D. Moran, S. Balasubramanyan, and P.A. Smith. "Effects and Consequences of Nerve Injury on the Electrical Properties of Sensory Neurons." *Can J Physiol Pharmacol.* 2003 Jul;81(7): pp. 663–82.

Altman, R.D. "A Rationale for Combining Acetaminophen and NSAIDs for Mild-to-moderate Pain." *Clin Exp Rheumatol.* 2004 Jan–Feb;22(1): pp. 110–7.

Apkarian, A.V., M.C. Bushnell, R.D. Treede, and J.K. Zubieta. "Human Brain Mechanisms of Pain Perception and Regulation in Health and Disease." *Eur J Pain.* 2005 Aug;9(4): pp. 463–84.

Arendt-Nielsen, L.P. Bajaj, A.M. Drewes. "Visceral Pain: Gender Differences in Response to Experimental and Clinical Pain." *Eur J Pain.* 2004 Oct;8(5): pp. 465–72.

Audette, J.F., E. Emenike, and A.L. Meleger. "Neuropathic Low Back Pain." *Curr Pain Headache Rep.* 2005 Jun;9(3): pp. 168–77.

Barbara, G., R. De Giorgio, V.Stanghellini, C. Cremon, B. Salvioli, and R. Corinaldesi. "New Pathophysiological Mechanisms in Irritable Bowel Syndrome." *Aliment Pharmacol Ther.* 2004 Jul;20 Suppl 2: pp. 1–9.

Benabid, A.L., B.Wallace, J. Mitrofanis, C. Xia, B. Piallat, V. Fraix, A. Batir, P. Krack, P. Pollak, and F. Berger. "Therapeutic Electrical Stimulation of the Central Nervous System." *C R Biol.* 2005 Feb;328(2): pp. 177–86.

Blackshaw, L.A., and G.F. Gebhart. "The Pharmacology of Gastrointestinal Nociceptive Pathways." *Curr Opin Pharmacol.* 2002 Dec;2(6): pp. 642–9.

Bloodworth, D. "Issues in Opioid Management." *Am J Phys Med Rehabil.* 2005 Mar;84(3 Suppl): pp. 42–55.

Borsook, D. "Pain: The Past, Present and Future." *Adv Drug Deliv Rev.* 2003 Aug 28;55(8): pp. 931–4.

Broadman, L.M. "Non-steroidal Anti-inflammatory Drugs, Antiplatelet Medications and Spinal Axis Anesthesia." *Best Pract Res Clin Anaesthesiol.* 2005 Mar;19(1): pp. 47–58.

Campbell, J.N. "Nerve Lesions and the Generation of Pain." *Muscle Nerve.* 2001 Oct;24(10): pp. 1261–73.

Carragee, E.J. "Clinical Practice. Persistent Low Back Pain." *N Engl J Med.* 2005 May 5;352(18): pp. 1891–8 Review.

Cervero, F., and J.M. Laird. "Understanding the Signaling and Transmission of Visceral Nociceptive Events." *J Neurobiol.* 2004 Oct;61(1): pp. 45–54.

Christo, P.J., T.S. Grabow, and S.N. Raja. "Opioid Effectiveness, Addiction, and Depression in Chronic Pain." *Adv Psychosom Med.* 2004;25: pp. 123–37.

Collins, S.D., and I.P. Chessell. "Emerging Therapies for Neuropathic Pain." *Expert Opin Emerg Drugs.* 2005 Feb;10(1): pp. 95–108.

Cortelli, P., and G. Pierangeli. "Chronic Pain-autonomic Interactions." *Neurol Sci.* 2003 May;24 Suppl 2:S68–70.

Crowell, M.D., M.P. Jones, L.A. Harris, T.N. Dineen, V.A. Schettler, and K.W. Olden. "Antidepressants in the Treatment of Irritable Bowel Syndrome and Visceral Pain Syndromes." *Curr Opin Investig Drugs.* 2004 Jul;5(7): pp. 736–42.

Devor, M. "Unexplained Peculiarities of the Dorsal Root Ganglion." *Pain.* 1999 Aug;Suppl 6:S27–35.

Dieppe, P.A., and L.S. Lohmander. "Pathogenesis and Management of Pain in Osteoarthritis." *Lancet.* 2005 Mar 12;365(9463): pp. 965–73.

Duncan, G. "Mind-body Dualism and the Biopsychosocial Model of Pain: What Did Descartes Really Say?" *J Med Philos.* 2000 Aug;25(4): pp. 485–513.

Eshkevari, L. "Acupuncture and Pain: A Review of the Literature." *AANA J.* 2003 Oct;71(5): pp. 361–70.

Fajardo, M., and P.E. Di Cesare. "Disease-modifying Therapies for Osteoarthritis: Current Status." *Drugs Aging.* 2005;22(2): pp. 141–61.

Falci, S., L. Best, R. Bayles, D. Lammertse, and C. Starnes. "Dorsal Root Entry Zone Microcoagulation for Spinal Cord Injury-related Central Pain: Operative Intramedullary Electrophysiological Guidance and Clinical Outcome." *J Neurosurg.* 2002 Sep;97(2 Suppl): pp. 193–200.

Finger, Stanley. *Origins of Neuroscience: A History of Explorations into Brain Function.* New York: Oxford University Press, 1994.

Finnerup, N.B., and T.S. Jensen. "Spinal Cord Injury Pain—Mechanisms and Treatment." *Eur J Neurol.* 2004 Feb;11(2): pp. 73–82.

Flor, H. "Remapping Sensory Cortex After Injury." *Adv Neurol.* 2003;93: pp. 195–204.

Fricton, J.R. "The Relationship of Temporomandibular Disorders and Fibromyalgia: Implications for Diagnosis and Treatment." *Curr Pain Headache Rep.* 2004 Oct;8(5): pp. 355–63.

Gallagher, R.M. "Rational Integration of Pharmacologic, Behavioral, and Rehabilitation Strategies in the Treatment of Chronic Pain." *Am J Phys Med Rehabil.* 2005 Mar;84(3 Suppl):S64–76.

Giller, C.A. "The Neurosurgical Treatment of Pain." *Arch Neurol.* 2003 Nov;60(11): pp. 1537–40.

Greer, K.R., and J.W. Hoyt. "Pain: Theory, Anatomy, and Physiology." *Crit Care Clin.* 1990 Apr;6(2): pp. 227–34.

Han, J.S. "Acupuncture and Endorphins." *Neurosci Lett.* 2004 May 6;361(1–3): pp. 258–61.

Hansen, G.R., and J. Streltzer. "The Psychology of Pain." *Emerg Med Clin North Am.* 2005 May;23(2): pp. 339–48.

Holden, J.E., and J.A. Pizzi. "The Challenge of Chronic Pain." *Adv Drug Deliv Rev.* 2003 Aug 28;55(8): pp. 935–48.

Hulsebosch, C.E. "From Discovery to Clinical Trials: Treatment Strategies for Central Neuropathic Pain After Spinal Cord Injury." *Curr Pharm Des.* 2005;11(11): pp. 1411–20.

Huntley, A.L., J.T. Coon, and E. Ernst. "Complementary and Alternative Medicine for Labor Pain: A Systematic Review." *Am J Obstet Gynecol.* 2004 Jul;191(1): pp. 36–44.

Jage J. "Opioid Tolerance and Dependence—Do They Matter?" *Eur J Pain.* 2005 Apr;9(2): pp. 157–62.

Jasmin, L., M.V. Wu, and P.T. Ohara. "GABA Puts a Stop to Pain." *Curr Drug Targets CNS Neurol Disord.* 2004 Dec;3(6): pp. 487–505.

Kandel, Eric R., and James H. Schwarz. *Principles of Neural Science.* New York: Elsevier, 1985.

Kanpolat, Y. "The Surgical Treatment of Chronic Pain: Destructive Therapies in the Spinal Cord." *Neurosurg Clin N Am.* 2004 Jul;15(3): pp. 307–17.

Keefe, F.J., A.P. Abernethy, and L. Campbell. "Psychological Approaches to Understanding and Treating Disease-related Pain." *Annu Rev Psychol.* 2005;56: pp. 601–30.

Lee, Y., C. Rodriguez, and R.A. Dionne. "The Role of COX–2 in Acute Pain and the Use of Selective COX–2 Inhibitors for Acute Pain Relief." *Curr Pharm Des.* 2005;11(14):pp. 1737–55.

Meglio, M. "Spinal Cord Stimulation in Chronic Pain Management." *Neurosurg Clin N Am.* 2004 Jul;15(3): pp. 297–306.

Melzack, R. "Pain: The Past, Present and Future." *Can J Exp Psychol.* 1993 Dec;47(4): pp. 615–29.

Middleton, C. "The Causes and Treatments of Phantom Limb Pain." *Nurse Times.* 2003 Sep 2–8;99(35): pp. 30–3.

Mollereau, C., M. Roumy, and J.M. Zajac. "Opioid-modulating Peptides: Mechanisms of Action." *Curr Top Med Chem.* 2005;5(3): pp. 341–55.

Nadler, S.F. "Nonpharmacologic Management of Pain." *J Am Osteopath Assoc.* 2004 Nov;104(11 Suppl 8):S6–12.

Nampiaparampil, D.E., and R.H. Shmerling. "A Review of Fibromyalgia." *Am J Manag Care.* 2004 Nov;10(11 Pt 1): pp. 794–800.

Offenbaecher, M., and M. Ackenheil. "Current Trends in Neuropathic Pain Treatments with Special Reference to Fibromyalgia." *CNS Spectr.* 2005 Apr;10(4): pp. 285–97.

Ohara, P.T., J.P. Vit, and L. Jasmin. "Cortical Modulation of Pain." *Cell Mol Life Sci.* 2005 Jan;62(1): pp. 44–52.

Pattinson, D., and M. Fitzgerald. "The Neurobiology of Infant Pain: Development of Excitatory and Inhibitory Neurotransmission in the Spinal Dorsal Horn." *Reg Anesth Pain Med.* 2004 Jan–Feb;29(1): pp. 36–44.

Penn, R.D. "Intrathecal Medication Delivery." *Neurosurg Clin N Am.* 2003 Jul;14(3): pp. 381–7.

Peterson, J. "Understanding Fibromyalgia and Its Treatment Options." *Nurse Pract.* 2005 Jan;30(1): pp. 48–55; quiz pp. 56–7.

Rawlings, C.E. 3rd, A.O. el-Naggar, and B.S. Nashold, Jr. "The DREZ Procedure: An Update on Technique." Br J Neurosurg. 1989;3(6): pp. 633-42.

Romanelli, P., V. Esposito, and J. Adler. "Ablative Procedures for Chronic Pain." *Neurosurg Clin N Am.* 2004 Jul;15(3): pp. 335–42.

Romo, R., A. Hernandez, E. Salinas, C.D. Brody, A. Zainos, L. Lemus, V. de Lafuente, and R. Luna. "From Sensation to Action." *Behav Brain Res.* 2002 Sep 20;135(1–2): pp. 105–18.

Romo, R., and E. Salinas. "Touch and Go: Decision-making Mechanisms in Somatosensation." *Annu Rev Neurosci.* 2001;24: pp. 107–37.

Ross, E. "The Management of Pain in Arthritis and the Use of Cyclooxygenase-2 Inhibitors: New Paradigms and Insights." *Curr Pain Headache Rep.* 2004 Dec;8(6): pp. 518–22.

Rushton, D.N. "Electrical Stimulation in the Treatment of Pain." *Disabil Rehabil.* 2002 May 20;24(8): pp. 407–15.

Sachs, C.J. "Oral Analgesics for Acute Nonspecific Pain." *Am Fam Physician.* 2005 Mar 1;71(5): pp. 913–8.

Sandkuhler, J., and R. Ruscheweyh. "Opioids and Central Sensitisation: I. Preemptive Analgesia." *Eur J Pain.* 2005 Apr;9(2): pp. 145–8.

Schaible, H.G., A. Del Rosso, and M. Matucci-Cerinic. "Neurogenic Aspects of Inflammation." *Rheum Dis Clin North Am.* 2005 Feb;31(1): pp. 77–101, ix.

Smith, P.A. "Neuropathic Pain: Drug Targets for Current and Future Interventions." *Drug News Perspect.* 2004 Jan–Feb;17(1): pp. 5–17.

Starkstein, S.E., and R.G. Robinson. "Mechanism of Disinhibition After Brain Lesions." *J Nerv Ment Dis.* 1997 Feb;185(2): pp. 108–14.

Staud, R. "Fibromyalgia Pain: Do We Know the Source?" *Curr Opin Rheumatol.* 2004 Mar;16(2): pp. 157–63.

Suzuki, R., L.J. Rygh, and A.H. Dickenson. "Bad News From the Brain: Descending 5-HT Pathways That Control Spinal Pain Processing." *Trends Pharmacol Sci.* 2004 Dec;25(12): pp. 613–7.

Vanegas, H., and H.G. Schaible. "Descending Control of Persistent Pain: Inhibitory or Facilitatory?" *Brain Res Rev.* 2004 Nov;46(3): pp. 295–309.

Wallace, B.A., K. Ashkan, and A.L. Benabid. "Deep Brain Stimulation for the Treatment of Chronic, Intractable Pain." *Neurosurg Clin N Am.* 2004 Jul;15(3): pp. 343–57.

Warner, T.D., and J.A. Mitchell. "Cyclooxygenases: New Forms, New Inhibitors, and Lessons from the Clinic". *FASEB J.* 2004 May;18(7): pp. 790–804.

Waxman, S.G., S. Dib-Hajj, T.R. Cummins, and J.A. Black. "Sodium Channels and Pain." *Proc Natl Acad Sci USA.* 1999 Jul 6;96(14): pp. 7635–9.

Weiner, D.K., and E. Ernst. "Complementary and Alternative Approaches to the Treatment of Persistent Musculoskeletal Pain." *Clin J Pain.* 2004 Jul–Aug;20(4): pp. 244–55.

Weinstein, J. "Neurogenic and Nonneurogenic Pain and Inflammatory Mediators." *Orthop Clin North Am.* 1991 Apr;22(2): pp. 235–46.

Willis, William D. *Sensory Mechanisms of the Spinal Cord.* New York: Kluwer Academic/Plenum Publishers, 2004.

Wood, J.N. "Recent Advances in Understanding Molecular Mechanisms of Primary Afferent Activation." *Gut.* 2004 Mar;53 Suppl 2:ii9–12.

Woodhouse, A. "Phantom Limb Sensation." *Clin Exp Pharmacol Physiol.* 2005 Jan–Feb;32(1–2): pp. 132–4.

Woolf, C.J., and M. Costigan. "Transcriptional and Posttranslational Plasticity and the Generation of Inflammatory Pain." *Proc Natl Acad Sci USA.* 1999 Jul 6;96(14): pp. 7723–30.

Yezierski, R.P. "Pain Following Spinal Cord Injury: Pathophysiology and Central Mechanisms." *Prog Brain Res.* 2000;129: pp. 429–49.

Further Reading

Cameron, Oliver G. *Visceral Sensory Neuroscience: Interoception.* New York: Oxford University Press, 2002.

Casey, Kenneth L., ed. *Pain and Central Nervous System Disease: The Central Pain Syndromes.* Bristol-Myers Squibb Symposium on Pain Research, University of Michigan, 1990. New York: Raven Press, 1991.

Deyo R.A. "Low-back Pain." *Sci Am.* 1998 Aug;279(2): pp. 48–53.

Dyck, Peter James. *Peripheral Neuropathy.* Philadelphia: Saunders, 1993.

Foley, K.M. "Controlling the Pain of Cancer." *Sci Am.* 1996 Sep;275(3): pp. 164–5.

Kornhuber, H.H., ed. *The Somatosensory System.* Acton, Mass.: Publishing Sciences Group, 1975.

Meldrum, Marcia L. *Opioids and Pain Relief: A Historical Perspective.* Seattle, Wash.: IASP Press, 2003.

Melton, L. "Aching Atrophy: More Than Unpleasant, Chronic Pain Shrinks the Brain." *Sci Am.* 2004 Jan;290(1): pp. 22–4.

Melzack, R. "Phantom Limbs." *Sci Am.* 1992 Apr;266(4): pp. 120–6.

Melzack, R. "The Tragedy of Needless Pain." *Sci Am.* 1990 Feb;262(2): pp. 27–33.

Morris, David B. *The Culture of Pain.* Berkeley: University of California Press, 1991.

Pace, J. Blair. *Pain: A Personal Experience.* Chicago: Nelson-Hall, 1976.

Rist, Curtis. "The Pain Is in the Brain." *Discover,* 21, no. 3 (2000).

Rosenthal, Elisabeth. "The Pain Game." *Discover,* 14, no. 11 (1993).

Stix, G. "A Toxin Against Pain." *Sci Am.* 2005 Apr;292(4): pp. 70–5.

Wall, Patrick D., and Ronald Melzack, eds. *Textbook of Pain.* Edinburgh and New York: Churchill Livingstone, 1999.

Web Sites

A Brief History of Pain
   http://abcnews.go.com/Health/PainManagement/
   story?id=731553&page=1

How You Feel Pain
   http://www.mayoclinic.com/invoke.cfm?id=PN00017

Pain Control
   http://www.cancersupportivecare.com/pain.html

Pain Disorders
   http://familydoctor.org/x5412.xml

Pain Research
   http://www.niams.nih.gov/hi/topics/pain/pain.htm

The Skin
   http://faculty.washington.edu/chudler/receptor.html

Spinal Cord Injury—Christopher Reeve Paralysis Foundation
   http://www.christopherreeve.org/

The Whole Brain Atlas
   http://www.med.harvard.edu/AANLIB/home.htm

Picture Credits

Index

About the Author

Bryan C. Hains, Ph.D., began his academic training at Stetson University (B.S., Biology) and then studied at Boston University (M.A., Neurobiology), the University of Texas Medical Branch (Ph.D., Neuroscience), and Yale University (post-doctoral training). Still in New Haven, he is currently an Assistant Professor of Neurology and conducts research on nerve injury and pain within the Center for Neuroscience and Regeneration Research at Yale University.

About the Editor

Eric H. Chudler, Ph.D., is a research neuroscientist who has investigated the brain mechanisms of pain and nociception since 1978. He is currently a research associate professor in the University of Washington Department of Bioengineering and director of education and outreach at University of Washington Engineered Biomaterials. Dr. Chudler's research interests focus on how areas of the central nervous system (cerebral cortex and basal ganglia) process information related to pain. He has also worked with other neuroscientists and teachers to develop educational materials to help students learn about the brain.